DELIVERED BY MIDWIVES

DELIVERED BY
MIDWIVES

*African American Midwifery
in the Twentieth-Century South*

JENNY M. LUKE

UNIVERSITY PRESS OF MISSISSIPPI / JACKSON

www.upress.state.ms.us

Designed by Peter D. Halverson

The University Press of Mississippi is a member of the
Association of University Presses.

First printing 2018

∞

Library of Congress Cataloging-in-Publication Data

Names: Luke, Jenny M., 1965– author.
Title: Delivered by midwives : African American midwifery in the twentieth-
century South / Jenny M. Luke.
Description: Jackson : University Press of Mississippi, [2018] | Includes biblio-
graphical references and index. |
Identifiers: LCCN 2018017426 (print) | LCCN 2018018619 (ebook) | ISBN
9781496818928 (epub single) | ISBN 9781496818935 (epub instititional) | ISBN
9781496818942 (pdf single) | ISBN 9781496818959 (pdf institutional) | ISBN
9781496818911 (cloth : alk. paper) | ISBN 9781496821133 (pbk. : alk. paper)
Subjects: LCSH: African American midwives—Southern States—History—
20th century. | Midwifery—Southern States—History—20th century. |
Childbirth—History—20th century.
Classification: LCC RG950 (ebook) | LCC RG950 .L85 2018 (print) | DDC
618.20089/96075—dc23
LC record available at https://lccn.loc.gov/2018017426

British Library Cataloging-in-Publication Data available

IN RECOGNITION OF THE WORK AND DEDICATION OF AFRICAN AMERICAN
LAY MIDWIVES IN THE TWENTIETH-CENTURY SOUTH

CONTENTS

ACKNOWLEDGMENTS IX
INTRODUCTION 3

PART 1. Motherwit: Lay Midwifery 13

CHAPTER 1. Out of Slavery 17
CHAPTER 2. Cultural Motifs Persist 25
CHAPTER 3. Licensing and the "New Laws" 32
CHAPTER 4. Implementing the Changes 39
CHAPTER 5. Working with the State 52
CHAPTER 6. Working with Physicians 59

PART 2. Asafetida to Aureomycin: African American Nurse-Midwives . . 63

CHAPTER 7. Establishing the Professional Nurse-Midwife 67
CHAPTER 8. African American Nurse-Midwives 73
CHAPTER 9. The Application of Nurse-Midwives 83
CHAPTER 10. Problems of Racism and Challenges to Professionalism . . 91

PART 3. Changing Attitudes and Better Access 95

CHAPTER 11. Overcoming Challenges 97
CHAPTER 12. African American Women Turn to Hospital Birth 109
CHAPTER 13. Changing Childbirth Customs 118

PART 4. Midwifery in Transition 121

CHAPTER 14. Lay Midwives "Retire" 125
CHAPTER 15. Midwifery Becomes a White Woman's Realm 133
CHAPTER 16. Midwifery Today and Its Potential for Tomorrow 138

CONTENTS

EPILOGUE 145
NOTES 151
BIBLIOGRAPHY 176
INDEX 189

ACKNOWLEDGMENTS

When I began researching midwifery it was never my intention to write a book. My interest was piqued twenty-seven years ago when I arrived in the United States from Britain and discovered that Americans perceived my work as a nurse-midwife very differently than did Britons; it was as a student of American history that I became fascinated. The evolution of the book was piecemeal, each intermediary step forward coming at the encouragement and guidance of several important individuals.

For many years I received generous support and recognition from the history faculty at the University of Texas at Arlington, in particular Stephanie Cole, Elisabeth Cawthon, and Christopher Morris, who nurtured my growth as a historian and saw potential in my work and me. It was at their prompting that I continued my research, and I would like to express my sincere gratitude to them. I am especially thankful for Stephanie Cole. As I navigated an unfamiliar world of publication, her practical advice was invaluable, as was her scholarly expertise in the field of race and gender in the South.

I am fortunate to have received support from a number of archives and institutions that enabled me to complete this book; their financial assistance made research trips feasible. I would like to thank the Waring Library Society and the Waring Historical Library at the Medical University of South Carolina for acknowledging my research with the W. Curtis Worthington Jr. prize. One element of the award is publication in the *Journal of the South Carolina Medical Association*; however, my essay "Asafetida to Aureomycin: African American Nurse-Midwives, 1930–1950" was never published. The journal declared a conflict of interest was at the crux of its refusal, but the decision reinforced the relevance of the topic and gave me confidence to pursue further research. I am grateful to Susan Hoffius, curator of the Waring Library, for her help in facilitating my visit there. I am indebted to Peggy Balch at the Reynolds-Finley Historical Library and Tim Pennycuff at the University of Alabama at Birmingham Archives for their assistance during my brief but productive stint at the Lister Hill Library as a Reynolds-Finley fellow. Both were tremendously helpful and expertly anticipated my research needs; it was a pleasure to work with them. I thank them for their continued support and their prompt response to my many e-mailed queries on source material.

I extend my sincere appreciation to William Thompson, who helped me plow through a great quantity of material during a time-constrained visit to the Mississippi Department of Archives and History in Jackson, and to Barrye Brown of the Avery Research Center at the College of Charleston for her assistance with the Dr. Elizabeth M. Bear Collection and for guiding me toward other potential sources. I thank her for her genuine interest in my work.

This exercise in historical research is made more relevant by professional insight, and I am grateful for the input of Dr. Helen Barnes and certified nurse-midwives Joselyn Bacon, Heather Clarke, and Lesley Rathbun. Their perspective as maternity care providers enabled me to make connections between the past and the present, and each gave their precious time generously. My particular thanks go to Dr. J. Edward Hill, whose forthcoming retirement will be an enormous loss to the medical profession, such is his commitment to equitable health care; it was a privilege to meet him and I look forward to reading his memoir now that he has time to turn his attention to writing. Winifred Connerton of the archive committee at the American College of Nurse-Midwives was instrumental in affording me access to many of the images included in the book, and I appreciate her assistance.

The University Press of Mississippi has expertly converted my manuscript into book form via the usual process of anonymous reader reviews, revisions, and copyediting, and I thank Craig Gill and Katie Keene among others for their guidance. I fondly remember Katie patiently answering my many (probably very simplistic) questions over a fabulous Mississippi-style breakfast in Jackson. Her kind reassurance alleviated any anxieties I had. Although I accepted all assistance offered, any errors are mine alone.

Finally, I must recognize my wonderful family and friends on both sides of the Atlantic who have shown absolute delight in my success; without their support and encouragement I would have turned back at the first hurdle. I cannot thank them enough, and I look forward to a time when I do not subject them to conversations that somehow always revert to midwifery or "the book."

DELIVERED BY MIDWIVES

INTRODUCTION

In each community, large or small, the essential problem is the same—how to bring about a general realization of the need for adequate care for each woman at childbirth and how to secure such care.

GRACE L. MEIGS, CHILDREN'S BUREAU, 1917

"I got so much experience in here I just want to explode . . . I want somebody to realize what I am," exclaimed Onnie Lee Logan toward the end of her life as she voiced her demand to be heard, to be given the opportunity to share her experience and knowledge.[1] As a lay midwife in Alabama, she devoted her life to improving the health of her community and was recognized for such in 1989, when the mayor of Mobile announced a local holiday in her honor: Onnie Lee Logan Day. Across the state in Eutaw, her seventy-nine-year-old counterpart, Margaret Charles Smith, was the first African American to be awarded the key to the city; she too was celebrated with an eponymous holiday. Until midwifery was declared illegal in the late 1970s, thousands of lay midwives like Mrs. Smith and Mrs. Logan were the sole providers of maternity care to generations of southern women.[2] Only a few of these elderly African American women were acknowledged for their steadfast commitment to a service that was once essential, but came to be considered surplus to requirements. However, in 2009, at an event dedicated to the legendary Margaret Charles Smith, the *Birmingham Weekly* newspaper quoted Jennifer Crook Moore lamenting the fact that for many poor women access to maternity care was still desperately inadequate. She exclaimed, "There are ten counties in the Black Belt, and ten of them have no hospital maternity services . . . it's just baffling. And those are the areas where the midwives used to work."[3] Moore's point speaks to a wider truth than she implied. Data gathered by the government-supported Southern Rural Black Women's Initiative (SRBWI) shines a harsh spotlight on the appalling lack of care for women in the rural South. In almost every social indicator

3

of well-being—poverty, income and employment, education, health, public infrastructure and housing—the rural counties of the South's Black Belt across Georgia, Alabama, and Mississippi are identified as some of the most neglected in the United States. Jennifer Crook Moore's protest of almost a decade ago remains a bitter reality today as fewer than one-half of women in the rural South live within a thirty-minute drive of the nearest clinic or hospital offering maternity services.[4]

In roughly a century a few landmark moments shifted the availability of maternal health care to poor, black women. With the passage of the Sheppard-Towner Maternity and Infancy Act in 1921, government regulation and supervision of midwifery began; at the time, midwifery was the most prominent form of maternity care for African American women in the South. With civil rights legislation and the integration of hospitals, access to the medical establishment widened, and the implementation of Medicaid later in the 1960s brought modern maternity care within reach of the economically vulnerable. However, if the current maternal and infant mortality figures are any indication, another landmark shift is long overdue. The history of medicine has generally been studied with the assumption that scientific progress, in this case the medicalization of childbirth, is linear, unidirectional, and always positive. Although it is foolish to deny the proven benefits of modern medicine, the "things-are-getting-better-all-the-time" approach must be recognized for its failings and the current trend in maternity care validates this perspective.

The maternal and infant mortality rate is the equivalent of a report card with regard to the wholesale quality of maternity care, and when compared to the national rates of countries with similar economies, the United States has a failing grade despite consistently outspending its peers. To put it in perspective, between 2003 and 2013, the United States was one of eight countries, and the only developed one in a group that includes South Sudan and Afghanistan, where maternal mortality is rising, and US women are at a higher risk of dying than those giving birth in China or Saudi Arabia.[5] Moreover, African American women are three times as likely to die from pregnancy-related complications than are white women, and black infant mortality is more than twice as high.

The provision of effective maternity care is far more than simply ensuring the presence of a suitably qualified attendant at birth; early and consistent care throughout pregnancy is central to lowering mortality. When interviewed by CNN, Dr. Andreea Creanga of the Center for Disease Control and Prevention (CDC) explained: "We know that black women dying from

pregnancy-related causes are younger, less educated, more likely to be unmarried, more likely to start prenatal care in the second [or] third trimester
of pregnancy, or not at all, when compared to white women, but except for
that, we don't know a lot."[6] The young, uneducated, and isolated mothers
profiled in the SRBWI study fit this description precisely, but black women
across the nation are at higher risk.

The situation is indeed at crisis point and legislators in Washington, DC,
have been presented with the Improving Access to Maternity Care Act of
2015, a bipartisan bill proposing to reimburse maternity care professionals in
return for their service in specifically identified regions of shortage, mainly
in rural areas. Passed by the House of Representatives and introduced in
the Senate in March 2017 the bill remains in the hands of the Committee on
Health, Education, Labor, and Pensions. The proposal highlights the simple
fact that the number of medical school graduates entering obstetrics-gyne-
cology (OB/GYN) has not significantly changed for three decades despite a
population increase of almost 25 percent.[7] It is little wonder then, that in 2011,
46 percent of US counties had no OB/GYN, and 40 percent of counties had
neither a certified nurse-midwife nor an OB/GYN.[8] Moreover, the American Congress of Obstetricians and Gynecologists (ACOG) has predicted a
shortfall of obstetricians to be around 9,000 by 2030.[9] In order to reverse the
rising trend of maternal and infant mortality a new approach must be found.

Ironically, solutions for the future may come to light by looking at maternity care for African American women over the last century. A useful backdrop against which to study maternity care is the Deep South, a subregion
of the South that includes the Carolinas, parts of Florida, Georgia, Alabama,
Mississippi, and Louisiana, where a legacy of midwifery endured and was
deeply ingrained in the culture. During most of the twentieth century, the
unique political, social, and economic climate of the Deep South forced a
reliance on African American lay midwives who served their communities
diligently. There are also some geographical outliers beyond the officially
designated borders of the Deep South, where isolated black populations were
large enough to sustain a midwifery-based childbirth culture. East Texas and
the remote Chesapeake coastline of eastern Virginia are culturally similar
if not physically part of the Deep South, and for the purposes of this book
they will be included in a more culturally defined Deep South.

By blending a modern understanding of health and well-being with a
more traditional, locally embedded, community-oriented model of maternal
health, we may gain guidance for improving maternity care and access today.
As Dr. J. Edward Hill, a former president of the American Medical Association

(AMA), asserted in 2006: "All health care is local. And, when folks at the local level get moving, they solve their problems." Progress does not always have to percolate down from the top; it can bubble up from the bottom.[10]

Dr. Collins Airhihenbuwa, a biobehavioral health specialist, promotes a cultural-empowerment model of health care as a way to address the significant health disparities being faced by African American communities. His community-level approach takes into consideration micro and macro factors of care, both of which, he argues, are necessary for acceptable and effective health-care provision.[11] Airhihenbuwa's model defines the micro elements of health as those found at the grassroots level: community and individual knowledge of health; how health is understood, interpreted, and transmitted; and how religion and spirituality relate to health, illness, and treatment. Macro components of health care, defined at the state and federal level, include hospitals, medical professionals, and scientific knowledge (as opposed to micro-level empirical knowledge). Macro-level health care brings with it state and federal structures and the associated hierarchy, the potential for racism, and the presumed superiority of Western modern medicine. This micro-macro categorization is essential for understanding what elements of maternal health care have altered over the last century for African American women, what has worked, and what has failed.

The connection between culture and health is not new, and Airhihenbuwa cautions that some early health initiatives designed for specific communities have been counterproductive. Deficit models tend to identify negative behaviors related to culture and attempt to alter behavior without acknowledging the different cultural lens through which the practitioners view the community. In these cases, the practitioners fail to see the agency of the community to choose how, when, and if they will participate in the local health initiative. Instead, Airhihenbuwa promotes the cultural-empowerment model as superior for African Americans because of its focus on the positive aspects of the community. He argues that African Americans "have a rich heritage of surviving and sometimes thriving in hostile contexts" and much of their resilience is grounded in the community and the church. He asserts that faith-based and community programs are the most effective portals for health education and culturally appropriate interventions intended to eliminate health disparities.[12] Training health-care professionals in cultural competency may solve one component of a multifaceted problem, but in harnessing a legacy of resourcefulness and resilience from within the community a more complete solution to inequalities in health and well-being may be achieved.

A similar cultural-empowerment approach to maternity care developed in the Deep South decades before Airhihenbuwa described his model theoretically. A collaboration between licensed lay midwives, public health nurses, and nurse-midwives resulted in a balance between the micro and macro factors of health care; health-care professionals supported influential lay practitioners in the community and care was improved by standardization and supervision. This model of care took into consideration health beliefs and cultural attitudes at the community or micro level, while simultaneously functioning in an expanding macro level of state intervention. However, since maternity care, like all aspects of medicine, is embedded within a larger framework of society, pressures of systemic racism in the region, circumscribed gender roles, and issues of professionalism prevented the long-term existence of this model of care.

Elsewhere in the South, a different isolated population relied on midwifery services. In the Appalachian Mountains of Kentucky, Mary Breckinridge established the Frontier Nursing Service in 1925 where her team of mainly British-trained nurse-midwives introduced scientific maternity care in a fashion that was in direct opposition to the collaboration evolving in the Deep South. Despite advice to the contrary, Breckinridge adamantly opposed the supervision of local lay midwives whom she believed wholly inadequate. The Bureau of Maternal and Child Health denied her funding in light of the positive results that were being achieved in other parts of the South where "midwives were eager to learn everything offered to them and gratefully accepted all instructions."[13] (It is important to note that the stance taken by the government was not founded on a plan to ensure the long-term survival and expansion of midwifery, merely a pragmatic short-term solution to the national disgrace of high maternal mortality.) After this rejection, Breckinridge severed all ties with the government and spent much of her career seeking private financing for her project, which survives today as the Frontier Nursing University. Mary Breckinridge's memoir *Wide Neighborhoods* and Melanie Beals Goan's balanced biography of Breckinridge, *Mary Breckinridge: The Frontier Nursing Service and Rural Health in Appalachia*, emphasize the broader issues surrounding the twentieth-century transformation of health care such as professionalism, gender roles, and class status.

This brief introduction to Mary Breckinridge's work serves to contrast two subregions of the South and illuminate the focus of this study: the dimension that race played in maternity care. Mary Breckinridge chose the location of her service based on what she deemed the worthiness of the people in Appalachia. By virtue of their geographic isolation these "mountaineers" were pure-blooded Anglo-Saxons and because she considered them to be above average intellect, they were "of the greatest possible value" to a nation under attack from city dwelling immigrants and African Americans.[14] In garnering financial support for the Frontier Nursing Service, Breckinridge played into the climate of fear and hostility that fueled the nativist resurgence and the eugenics movement of the 1920s and 1930s. Donors responded to her romanticized impression of these racially pure, hard-working people who were "a key repository of traditional values," and gave willingly.[15] In working to fulfill her vision, Breckinridge faced obstacles rooted in the prevailing assumptions of class and gender as she and her nurses interacted with the Appalachian communities they served. Contemporary assumptions of professionalism and presumed medical hierarchy also served as a challenge to her nurses. However, they and the women they served were not exposed to the devastating barrier of race that African American women, lay midwives, and nurses encountered in other parts of the South.

The inherent racism of the South created a unique environment that allowed a very particular—and as I argue, quite modern and potentially useful—style of maternity care to emerge. The strengths and weaknesses of the care provided can be ascertained by deconstructing it into its micro and macro components. When viewed across a time line beginning in 1920 with the onset of regulation, history shows that the micro elements of care, such as distinctive themes of spirituality and communal knowledge of health delivered by familiar and trusted women, were superseded by science-based, macro-level care administered in facilities by culturally distant practitioners. The gradual replacement of the micro component with the macro systems of medicine brought untold relief to millions of Americans, both black and white. However, given the current maternal and infant mortality rates, something is amiss.

This book charts the shift from a predominance of micro-level care, to a micro/macro blend, to an emphasis on the macro; it may be visualized as a balancing scale, the left-hand tray representing the degree of micro-level care, the right-hand tray, macro-level care. One might expect the "sweet spot" to be at the midpoint, the point at which a balance of micro and macro components produce optimum maternity care. However, history informs us that reality is never so easily determined, though it may enlighten the future and frame emerging health-care policies. In keeping with the balancing scale analogy, the book is organized by style of care rather than chronology, as there is too much chronological overlap in the four broad sections. The first section begins by locating the history in its cultural context and identifying the unique cultural motifs of African American childbirth that crystallized during slavery, persisted through emancipation, and endured throughout our time period. In six chapters, the section explores the role of traditional lay midwives and how they adapted to the increasing presence of local, state, and federal public health mandates beginning in the early 1920s: how they interacted with county health officers and local physicians, how they overcame the disadvantages of poverty and a limited education to meet standards of practice mandated by the state, how they exerted their influence to become valuable assets to county health departments. Lay midwives expertly fulfilled the micro-level elements of care and gently molded childbirth culture into a more modern form, but they were limited in their efficacy by an inability to access macro-level care. A bridge to macro health care was created by the introduction of certified nurse-midwives in the 1940s and an exploration of the issues and surrounding debates follows in part 2. Chapters 7 through 10 address the reinforcement of micro-level care with the modern, scientific macro components so critical to minimizing maternal and infant mortality. There is a broad focus on the clash of philosophies of community-based midwifery care and the scientific Western model of obstetric care. Chapter 10 specifically highlights the challenges faced by African American nurses and nurse-midwives as they navigated a professional arena plagued by systemic racism at the macro level. Part 3 exposes the specific problems encountered by African American women in a maternity care system dominated by macro-level care. To provide some historical context on the available medical care and facilities in the region, chapter 11 explores the enormous obstacles negotiated by a small cadre of black physicians and acknowledges the presence of all-black hospital facilities prior to the integration of medicine in the mid-1960s. With physician-led, hospital-based pregnancy and childbirth a feasible option for African American women by the 1950s, chapters 12 and 13 explore the reality of their experience in a racially segregated hospital system. The final section, part 4, addresses the transitions in midwifery across our time period beginning in chapter 14 with the various ways in which lay midwives were phased out, initially by restrictions on licensing, and later by legislation. With lay midwifery on the wane, chapter 15 describes the more recent development of nurse-midwifery and the professional challenges faced in defining a space in which to practice within a medically dominated maternity care landscape. Part 4 ends with an overview of contemporary midwifery and presents some optimistic evidence to suggest that the legacy of African American midwifery is being rekindled to help reverse the disparity of outcome for black childbearing women and their babies. This section reiterates the centrality of early and effective prenatal care to high-quality maternity care. In an epilogue, I revisit the analogy of the balancing scales and use history to argue that a model of maternity care that utilizes micro and macro components is optimal, not at the balancing point, but rather when both are integrated in a holistic approach. In other words, when both aspects of care are considered valid parts of a whole, and one is not sacrificed for the sake of the other.

The collapse of African American lay midwifery has been well document-ed by the work of women's health activist, Linda Janet Holmes, anthropologist Gertrude Jacinta Fraser, and Debra Ann Susie among others. A handful of lay midwives preserved their experiences in the form of memoirs and oral histories, and the work of four such women, Onnie Lee Logan, Margaret Charles Smith, Claudine Curry Smith, and Gladys Milton, is the linchpin of this book. The physical role of these state-licensed lay midwives, and the actual care they provided has been overlooked in most studies in favor of a focus on their anthropological and societal function. The studies focus on the demise of midwifery as a black-versus-white issue, but this is an over-simplification of a complex shift in childbirth culture. It fails to account for the changing expectations and agency of African American women, their rejection of a two-tier maternity care system, or their demand to be part of an inclusive, desegregated society. The few professionally trained and educated African American nurse-midwives have been neglected too, perhaps because of the dearth of primary sources available. Beyond the valuable memoirs of the lay midwives, the bulk of historical sources on black midwifery are found in medical and nursing journals, on the pages of which the debates on health care were fought. It is through these voices of both the professionals and the lay practitioners that the childbirth experience of poor and voiceless African American women can be interpreted.

Much more has been written about the professionalization of midwifery in America. Unlike their Western European counterparts who were regu-lated and held in high esteem by a national maternity care system early in the twentieth century, American midwives of all ethnicities were faced with elimination. The overwhelming political strength of the medical estab-lishment and a competitive economic marketplace has inhibited American midwives' ability to establish themselves as legitimate providers of maternity care. This unique national narrative is detailed in the new encyclopedic *The History of Midwifery in the United States* written by two leaders in nurse-midwifery, Helen Varney Burst and Joyce Beebe Thompson. Laura Ettinger's *Nurse-Midwifery: The Birth of a New American Profession* presents a more nuanced history that encompasses a wider social context. Broader histories of childbearing in America include the 1970s and 1980s scholarship of Richard W. and Dorothy C. Wertz, Judith Walzer Leavitt, and Pamela S. Eakins, whose works coincided with a renewed understanding of childbirth as a female experience influenced by culture and choice. Reflecting the era's shift toward a less interventionist childbirth demanded by dissatisfied white middle- and upper-class women, these histories speak to the consumer demands that drive maternity care.

Along with the concepts of "micro" and "macro" care, the specific nomenclature relating to the various denominations of midwife needs to be clarified. Because midwifery is governed at the state level much variation exists in the classification. The narrative begins with lay midwives who, with no formal training or education, gained their knowledge by observation, and their skills developed by experience under an apprenticeship. Many became licensed by the state; however, this did not raise them to the status of certified nurse-midwives. Lay midwives in some sources are also referred to as granny midwives, but not all midwives were elderly so lay midwife seems to be a better term and will be used throughout. Certified nurse-midwives (CNM) are registered nurses with postgraduate education and clinical training specifically in the care of women. Nurse-midwives practice legally in all states, mainly in a hospital setting. Like CNMs, certified midwives (CM) are registered by the American College of Nurse-Midwives, but do not have a foundation in nursing; they are much fewer in number than CNMs, and only have legal status in three states. Some states allow the practice of certified professional midwives (CPM) who are independent practitioners certified by the North American Registry of Midwives, as are direct entry midwives (DEM) formally known as licensed (LM) or registered (RM) midwives. These categories of midwife do not have hospital privileges and are the only ones that require knowledge and experience of out-of-hospital settings. They are dwarfed in number by the more mainstream certified nurse-midwives. Varney and Thompson's *The History of Midwifery in the United States* provides an extensive description of midwifery credentialing.

The physiology of pregnancy and childbirth is unchanging and therefore acts as a constant that more readily exposes the shifting attitudes and accepted societal norms surrounding it. Rather than identifying trends and changes to enhance our understanding of the past, this book presents an opportunity not only to simply explore the childbirth experiences of the past, but also to look to history with a view to the future. Enabling women to have healthy babies after a safe pregnancy is more than "catchin' babies" as the midwives professed; it is as true a statement now as it was in the mid-decades of the twentieth century when aspects of lay midwifery were utilized so effectively.

This book takes a perspective that exposes the value of community-centered, culturally appropriate, holistic care once discarded as archaic and backward that may have actually solved health-care needs much better than the wholesale regulation that came later would suggest. Moreover, it provides an opportunity to focus on black midwives, particularly the lay midwives, a group of women who proved themselves to be pragmatic in the face of adversity, and ready to adapt and compromise as necessary. More often than not they impressed their superiors on a personal level, despite being collectively undervalued. They never lost sight of their objective to serve their communities to the best of their ability, and their unfaltering dignity and pride ultimately led them to personal triumph albeit at the expense of their own authority. An acknowledgment of the value of their work, and an attempt to rehabilitate some of the most effective aspects of their role suitably honors their lives.

Having introduced the scope, themes, and objective of this book, allow me to be clear about what it is not. This study of African American midwifery and maternity care is by no means a clarion call for a return to home birth and undereducated, inadequately trained midwives, far from it. As a British-trained nurse-midwife I am a staunch advocate of standards and regulation, and a firm proponent of midwifery as part of a multidisciplinary health-care team. Neither is it my intention to make a political stance, nor to propose policy. However, as the old adage goes, those who fail to learn from history are doomed to repeat it, and today, after a century of federal regulation of maternity care, the United States is once more disgraced by its national maternal mortality figures. I argue that by taking a pragmatic approach we may learn important lessons from what the past suggests for our current health-care dilemmas. Having not practiced midwifery for twenty-five years, I write from the perspective of a historian, and hope that if nothing else this book helps to preserve and promote the legacy of African American midwifery. As Maria Milton, a licensed midwife in the Florida Panhandle, explained, African Americans need to know their own history. This in itself holds the potential to enhance self-worth, restore faith in personal ability, and inspire communities.[16]

PART 1

MOTHERWIT

Lay Midwifery

The sun wasn't shinin' every time and the moon wasn't either. . . .
lateness of the hour or the earlies of the mornin' didn't bother me. I
just went when I was called. There has been a many dreary nights but
I didn't look at 'em as dreary nights. I had on my mind where I was
goin' and what I was goin' for.

ONNIE LEE LOGAN, 1989

"White doctors weren't too kind to us black folks," lay midwife Onnie Lee
Logan remembered, but it was not always lack of attention that prompted
her to come to this conclusion. In her personal experience of white doctors,
neglect was certainly a central feature, as she did not remember a single
incidence where a white doctor delivered a black baby in the home of the
mother. In fact, she joked that in an emergency situation "if they sent for him
[the doctor] the baby woulda been there and probably some of 'em walkin'
befo' he got there."[1] Onnie Lee Logan's impression of white doctors was probably modified for the better by her interaction with them as a state-licensed
midwife, but generally speaking many African American women in the Jim
Crow South had no expectation of medical care for pregnancy and childbirth.
Moreover, they were suspicious of the motivation of white physicians and
had little confidence in their skill and knowledge. The profound level of
distrust did not have its origins in neglect, but rather in the dehumanized
attention given to enslaved women by doctors during slavery. Doctors, at
the behest of slave owners, attempted to manage slave women's sexuality,
fertility, and childbirth with a view to increasing the slave owner's labor
pool and profitability, ultimately sustaining the "peculiar institution." This
scrutiny while in bondage and the subsequent neglect following emancipation shaped African American childbirth expectations and culture. There

was a duality in the knowledge of health in the freed black community; on one hand, they emerged from slavery with an arsenal of herbal remedies and healing treatments, and on the other, a clear comprehension of the potential danger of white medicine.[2] Any study of the maternity care of black women in America must be underpinned by a sound understanding of the culturally specific motifs that have persisted for generations. Furthermore, any attempt by health policy specialists to improve the disparity in the current maternity care system must be grounded in cultural awareness.

It seems odd that a group of poor, barely educated African American women, entirely powerless outside of their marginalized communities, would be the subject of vociferous debate in the professionalizing medical world, but so lay midwives were during the early decades of the twentieth century. Though maligned as "evil" and believed to undermine a physician's authority and right to economic security, these women were simply answering a vocational calling to serve their communities as generations of others had done before them. In the face of overwhelming poverty, deprivation, and systemic racial discrimination, they filled a void in the provision of care, and when incorporated into the long-term trajectory of maternity care during the twentieth century, lay midwifery was of immense value. Although the model of care was certainly deficient at the macro level given that access to professional scientific knowledge, medical expertise, and modern facilities was severely limited, the micro aspects of care were entirely fulfilled by these nonprofessional health-care providers who were embedded in the community they served.

Nevertheless, when viewed through the Eurocentric, patriarchic lens of a medical profession that placed scientific knowledge (macro level) above all other, they were dismissed as incompetent, obsolete, and dangerous. Added to this was a racial and gender bias that denigrated the intellectual capacity of African Americans and deemed them incapable of functioning independently. In short, it was determined that midwifery had to be terminated. However, with neither a financial incentive, nor any real inclination to assist poor black women, an immediate and complete eradication of black midwifery was unfeasible and a more pragmatic compromise was implemented. Through a process of regulation and supervision African American lay midwives were presented with an opportunity to enhance their knowledge in basic modern techniques, and as the slave midwives did before them, they integrated the newly acquired skills into their practice. Their history illuminates the complex dilemma that faced black lay midwives as they not only navigated the increasingly formalized health-care options, but also accommodated to the shifting cultural demands of the women they served. It was a double-edged sword: they were adamant that their micro-level skills were invaluable, and that the trusting, respectful relationships they had with their patients were critical, but simultaneously, they were instrumental in helping women gain access to modern, macro-level maternity care. In some respects, they were the victims of their own success.

CHAPTER 1

OUT OF SLAVERY

African slaves brought with them a concept of health and healing that melded in the crucible of slavery to produce a unique culture and understanding of health. Christianity was incorporated into West and West-Central African religious principles to produce what Sharla Fett has called a relational vision of health that connected individuals to the community, their ancestors, and faith. Illness could arise from neglected or contentious relationships between the living and the spirit world, and so slave healers and midwives were granted their authority to practice by their ability to transcend the real world into the spiritual realm. Their ability to do this was determined by their ancestry, spirituality, and witnessed skills. Both men and women were authorized to be healers; however, evidence suggests that most healers and midwives were women, typically older women. Given the nature of plantation work whereby male and younger female slaves were more likely to be assigned to physically strenuous work away from the immediate vicinity of the house, it seems reasonable that older women were responsible for attending the sick. Sickness was not something to be endured alone, and neither was healing possible without the consideration of extended social relationships. Midwives and healers were often granted a greater degree of mobility that enabled them to facilitate communication between family members and friends who may have been separated by sale or purchase.[1] The connection between individual and communal relationships in this vision of health bound the community tightly, bringing a sense of power and continuity in the face of enslavement. It was a power that the white medical establishment could not undermine.

The relational concept of health and healing came into direct conflict with the slave owners' notion of health that generally perceived slave healing to be quackery at best, and at worst a nonsensical superstition reflecting the diminished capacity of the African intellect. In contrast, white male physicians, employed at the behest of the slave owners, claimed their authority on scientific reason and knowledge that had been acquired through professional associations and reading medical journals.[2] Traditional knowledge gained by apprenticeship and empiricism was dismissed as ineffectual. Furthermore, racial and gender biases dictated that black women were considered incapable of being autonomous practitioners of healing. Unlike the communal vision of sickness, physicians saw illness from a purely biological standpoint and followed an interventionist approach, employing "heroic" treatments such as bloodletting and purging, the outcome of which was neither efficacious nor predictable. Their motivation for doing something rather than nothing came in the form of justification of their fee for service.

During the early and mid-nineteenth century, American medical theory did not definitively associate race and disease. Black and white health and sickness was perceived to be similar, albeit it with some differences in response to certain treatments. Vague statements published in medical journals, such as "the Caucasian seems to yield more readily to remedies than the African," led doctors to expect to encounter some "peculiarities" when treating black patients.[3] In fact, orthodox practice identified the conditions of slavery to be the key factor in black health, not biological race: poor housing, inadequate diet, overcrowding, and poor ventilation of homes. Couched in the absolute terms of white superiority over black, the difference between disease and illness in the enslaved and white population was a matter of degree not kind.[4] Therefore, a slave's susceptibility to a particular illness was interpreted as an indication of inferiority. In an era when medical practice was governed by the practical application and observed results of remedies, purges, and bleeding, antebellum physicians *did not* assign racial biology to black sickness. However, fully immersed in a slave-structured society, their conflation of race and slavery created space for the potential of an expansive biological racism. By the end of the nineteenth century, with institutionalized slavery no longer a feature of southern society, a scientific association between race and biology crystallized.[5]

The theoretical dichotomy between Western medical philosophy and the relational concept of health and healing is clear, but the two canons of knowledge did not function in isolated spheres of influence. Rather, historians have revealed areas of significant overlap illuminating a complexity of practice that is difficult to unravel. Under some circumstances it was in the best interest of the slave owner to exert his authority on plantation health, and slave healers were pragmatic enough to adopt Western medical treatments if they were proven to be effective. By the same token, a physician may incorporate a treatment from a healer or midwife if it was observed to be of benefit. However, in broad terms, a specific African American health culture developed and persisted under slavery and to some degree helped to mitigate the dehumanizing effects of objectifying black health. Moreover, it set in place cultural motifs that can be identified generations later. The association between spirituality, community, and wellness continued to cement community and ancestral bonds, and the acceptance of female authority in healing persisted long after the demise of slavery.

During the early decades of the nineteenth century, three seemingly unrelated events converged to alter the relationship between slaves, particularly female slaves, their owners, and physicians: the cessation of the importation of slaves, the western expansion of cotton, and a professionalizing medical establishment. In 1808 Congress ended America's participation in the international slave trade, and thereafter, the slave population could no longer be supplemented by importation. Consequently, as the US expanded westward and cotton production began to soar, it became increasingly important for the perpetuation of slavery and the profitability of cotton planters that slave women bore plenty of children; the enslaved female body became a means of production. A professionalizing medical establishment, and the nascent specialty of obstetrics and gynecology, provided a method by which the slave owners could achieve their goal. Between them, the concept of "soundness" materialized; a concept that married material property values and labor production to slave wellness. In other words, soundness was the relationship between the past, present, and potential health of a slave measured against his capacity to work.[6] For female slaves, soundness was also related to their ability to reproduce. A "sound" female slave was one who had proven fertility through the birth of a child and who was young enough to have many more. This concept was reflected in the market value of slaves: a "breeding woman" sold for $1,500, while a girl of fifteen who had no children and therefore had not yet proved her fertility sold for $800.[7]

The fact that the slave population could no longer be topped up by direct importation from Africa meant that the fecundity of women became a source of potential wealth for slave owners. A slave woman's successful pregnancy and childbirth was directly related to profit; the children of slaves would either enhance the labor force and profitability of the plantation, or they could be sold elsewhere. Slave owners approached the reproductive potential of their slaves in a businesslike way. The optimum situation with the greatest financial return was achieved when a slave woman performed the maximum amount of work and raised the maximum number of children. In reality, though, a balance had to be found so that the physical demands of slave work did not negatively impact her ability to carry a pregnancy to term. The renowned historian of slave health and medicine, Todd Savitt, asserts that in general, owners tended to indulge their women of childbearing age. He quotes Thomas Jefferson's order to an overseer not to coerce female workers into exerting themselves because "women are destroyed by exposure to wet at certain periodical indispositions to which nature has subjected them."[8] A successful slave-raising plantation raised the living conditions of slaves, kept the slaves well fed, and reduced the workload of menstruating women. Using this business model, a plantation in Mississippi reported a birth rate of 15 percent, twice the national average for slaves.[9] However, not all owners were so committed despite the potential for financial reward.

Owners tried to assert control over every aspect of enslaved women's reproductive lives. With the help of local doctors, they monitored the women's menstrual cycle and usually attempted to treat irregular menses with home remedies such as herbal or fruit teas. According to Savitt, disorders of menstruation and associated pain were widespread problems and the main cause of missed work, leading one physician in Virginia to remark that the loss of four to eight workdays per month was not unusual. The most common menstrual complaints were amenorrhea (the absence of menses), abnormal or irregular bleeding usually as a result of uterine fibroids or tumors, and abnormal discharge from conditions such as gonorrhea, tumors, and prolapsed uterus.[10] Some women used their owner's preoccupation with their fertility to advantage feigning an inability to work. An owner of numerous slaves complained about such malingering women: "The women on a plantation . . . will hardly earn their salt, after they come to the breeding age; they don't come to the field, and you go to the quarters and ask the old nurse what's the matter, and she says, 'oh, she's not well, master, she's not fit to work, sir': and what can you do? You have to take her word for it that something or other is the matter with her, and you dare not set her to work; and so she lays up until she feels like taking the air again, and plays the lady at your expense."[11]

Like their owners, slave women were also eager to regulate their menstrual cycles, but for different reasons: not so much to ensure their fertility, but to control it. One method of control was the use of cotton root as an emmenagogue, an agent that stimulates and regulates menstruation in women whose menstruation was absent for any reason, including pregnancy. That is not to say that a woman actively induced abortion; rather it was understood that there were many causes of amenorrhea, and if after using cotton root menses were not resumed, she understood herself to be pregnant. The shared knowledge, widespread availability, and ease of administration either by chewing or brewing into a tea, was a boon to women, enabling them to space their children as they so wished, but was of concern to slave owners who feared the loss of potential income. Marie Jenkins Schwartz succinctly describes the relationship between cotton, owners, and slave women: "The fortunes of slave holders rested on the portion of the plant that grew above ground, the destiny of women on the part below."[12] Physicians read about cotton root in their journals and many prescribed it as a treatment for their white patients, believing it to be safer and more effective than ergot. In 1852, a Dr. John Travis reported in the *Nashville Journal of Medicine and Surgery* that it "worked like a charm" in inducing menstruation.[13] It was one remedy in a physician's arsenal that was proven to be efficacious.

The designation of suitable sexual partners for maximum reproduction rates also fell into the domain of the slave owner. Former slaves recounted instances of forced sexual relationships, and Alabama midwife Margaret Charles Smith remembered that women of her grandmother's generation "had a certain man they had to marry when they got ready to marry because he had to be a breeding man."[14] The selective breeding at some plantations involved the allocation of four hand-picked slave women to one man selected for his good health and strength. A slave woman in Georgia described her treatment as similar to that of a brood sow.[15] Nonetheless, the formation and integrity of slave families, despite the intrusion of the slave owner, was crucial to survival, and community strength was rooted in kinship networks. Christopher Morris makes an insightful connection between master and slave families in his study of Warren County, Mississippi. By definition enslavement is dehumanizing, but he argues that masters "lived off, indeed they counted on, the very humanity of the people they oppressed."[16]

Although slave owners and some white physicians had suspicions about an excessive use of abortifacients by black women, enslaved people treasured motherhood, and ensuring the health of the unborn child presented slave women with a dilemma: reveal the pregnancy in the hope that they would receive a more nutritious diet and lighter work assignment or conceal it to avoid potentially dangerous interference from plantation physicians. In practice, though, pregnancy did not often result in a reduction in work demands or less risk of physical abuse, or in fact an improvement in diet. Neither did a white physician involve himself in every pregnancy. In most cases black midwives were relied upon to care for expectant slaves, and their elevated status allowed them to negotiate for better working and living conditions on the behalf of the women. As an example of the contradiction of plantation health care, there are many incidences of accommodations between black midwives and physicians. However, black health workers were seen as "sensible," "prudent," or "able" only within the context of physician supervision.[17] Plantation doctors never accepted the autonomous authority granted to black female health workers by their own community.

Slave women, of course, preferred to seek the advice of midwives and were more comfortable in their shared broad perception of health and wellness, with the familiar communal and religious components. Moreover, midwives were mothers both literally and symbolically; they were physical mothers of their own children, but the symbolic mother of each child they delivered, the mother of the community as they taught the skills of mothering, and the mother of a culture that was preserved and protected through generations of midwives.[18]

Their vital role garnered them power in the community to safely deliver cherished children, and with the slaveholder to safely increase his property value. However, it was a double-edged sword, as although slaveholders trusted them to some extent, enslaved midwives were generally considered capable of evading the direct orders of a physician. The midwives whose expanded realm of work also included caring for the sick and elderly were typically older women with an accumulation of experience, specialized knowledge, and a sense of autonomy that allowed them some freedom of judgment in the implementation of that knowledge. Although there is clear evidence that slave owners accepted the role of the midwife, and even on occasion sought her help for his own family, they rejected their spiritual empowerment as an authority to practice.[19]

Conflicts regarding practice generally came to a head at childbirth where there was the greatest potential for midwife and physician to work together. In all cultures, birth is a time of vulnerability for a woman and child, and the comforting rituals that govern the tasks carried out by trusted family members and attendants alleviate anxiety. Enslaved midwives provided these reassurances from their position at the center of the community. However, midwives straddled a line between the slave and slave owner. Her elevated position obligated her to call for a physician in the event of complications that usually included protracted labor, hemorrhage, convulsions, or cessation of contractions. Most midwives attempted to resolve the problem on their own, but if unable to rectify the issue, they were skeptical that the doctor was likely to do so either without loss of life. Physicians were eager for woman and child to survive, but since they were only called to difficult deliveries it is not surprising that slave women feared their attentions. Intervention by the physician was expected as they charged a fee for their expertise and were required to act. Furthermore, with their limited knowledge most treatments for obstetric emergencies were barbaric and often resulted in the loss of mother or baby or both. This interaction at childbirth reinforced the preference for the midwives' constant reassuring presence and seemingly timeless knowledge. To slaves, the physicians waited for a crisis and then attempted to manage it, running roughshod over their cherished rituals. For midwives, pragmatic as they were, this exposure to the larger medical world allowed them to observe and appraise techniques and incorporate them into their own practice if deemed to be helpful.

Many capable enslaved midwives earned a good reputation outside of their immediate plantation community and were often granted the freedom to attend women across the wider area, white women as well as black. What they gained in physical freedom of movement, they lost to some extent freedom of practice, as in order to maintain the trust of their owner they had to adhere to certain expectations. Having said that, the midwives who worked closely with the owners held more influence when negotiating for better conditions on behalf of the expectant slave women. Often the well-known midwives had had some level of apprenticeship with a physician. For example, Clara Walker was destined to become a midwife as she had fulfilled the traditional requirements by being born with "a veil on her face" permitting her greater spiritual awareness, but she was also apprenticed out to a physician and worked with him for five years.[20] Likewise, fifty-year-old Clarissa of South Carolina evidently spent some time working with a doctor. When being advertised for sale, her owner described her as "a first rate nurse and midwife; can be trusted to prescribe and mix physic."[21]

Although limited, the interchange of knowledge enhanced the enslaved midwives' ability to care for the women in their community, and some white physicians incorporated folk remedies into their practice. However, while white medicine focused narrowly on action and the treatment of specifics, the owners and physicians failed to recognize that the strength of slave healing lay not entirely in action but in the spirituality and authority of practitioners who were central to the broader community and culture. By creating a sacred health culture grounded in notions of authority that lay outside the realm of white society, the enslaved were able to preserve a relational vision of health that linked the well-being of an individual to the well-being of the community, and beyond to a spiritual life.[22]

The chaos and massive dislocation of newly freed slaves during the Civil War and Reconstruction severely tested the tenacity of black health culture. In fact, Jim Downs in his book, *Sick from Freedom*, asserts that the federal government's organization of freedpeople into a new system of forced labor "summarily stripped African Americans of their cultural resources to care for their bodies."[23] Inundated by the formerly enslaved, initially the Union army turned to the federal government for leadership, who in turn looked to local municipalities and private charitable groups for assistance. However, the enormity of meeting the health needs of a malnourished, sick, penniless, and homeless population was insurmountable. The federal response was to direct aid to areas of epidemic outbreak or documented need, but such an approach neglected huge swaths of the rural South where little assessment or documentation was undertaken.[24] Locally, municipal officials and almshouses generally refused to assist freedpeople because state and local governments failed to recognize them as citizens.[25] More locally still, former slave owners reneged on any obligation they felt toward meeting the health needs of black people. As one Louisiana planter crudely explained, "When I owned n******, I used to pay their medical bills and take care of them; I don't think I shall trouble myself much now."[26] As a new system of labor spread across the region, contracts between planters and laborers stipulated conditions of accommodation, land usage, equipment rental, and other necessities, but the responsibility for medical care was shifted entirely onto the worker.

Downs proposes that the failure of Reconstruction and the subsequent withdrawal of the federal government from the South had little impact on the health of African Americans because the initial intervention in the 1860s had never been successful. However, the withdrawal of physicians from childbirth allowed freedwomen the opportunity to regain control over their bodies, and they were free to handle pregnancy and childbirth according to their own notions of propriety.[27] As a result, midwives continued to support their isolated communities as best they could. The folk remedies initially brought from Africa, synthesized with Native American and some Western practices, persisted, and the necessity for self-reliance ensured that knowledge was consistently transmitted from one generation to the next. Self-help required a communal store of "motherwit," a blend of God-given wisdom and common sense that was usually in the possession of older women. It was into this childbirth culture and against this historical backdrop that government agencies, particularly the Children's Bureau, found themselves early in the twentieth century when once more, the federal government began to intervene in health care, this time specifically in maternal health.

CHAPTER 2

CULTURAL MOTIFS PERSIST

It was a 1917 publication by the federal Children's Bureau that triggered a governmental response to a national disgrace and brought midwifery into the crosshairs of debate. The report revealed an intolerably high maternal mortality rate and declared that the United States, when compared to sixteen other industrial countries, ranked fourteenth, with Spain and Belgium filling the bottom two places. Moreover, the study went on to reveal that the mortality rate for black women was double that of white women and that if accurate statistics from southern states were available, the disparity between the two groups would be magnified. This indicated "without a doubt" that there existed a "very great difference in standards of care at childbirth in these two groups."[1] For most in the medical profession, the responsibility for this disparity of care fell squarely on the shoulders of lay midwives. However, some physicians, recognizing the existence of a larger problem, challenged that assumption, arguing that "general practitioners lose as many and possibly more women from puerperal infection than do midwives."[2] A lackadaisical attitude to adopting newly accepted standards of medical practice prompted criticism from some in the profession. In urging an increased awareness of the importance of aseptic technique, Dr. W. C. Gewin wrote to the *Alabama Medical Journal*: "Among private practitioners there is still shown an adherence to antique methods which is to be greatly deplored. Why this should be is somewhat difficult to explain."[3] Compounding problems further was a physician's lack of clinical experience. As late as 1910, textbook and mannequins were relied upon as the sole teaching aids in medical schools, with few graduates ever having witnessed a birth. In the South, though, with its large African American population, few physicians, and its correspondingly high maternal mortality, midwifery was determined to be at the crux of the problem and lay midwives bore the brunt of the contempt.

By the 1920s most northern women, irrespective of social class and race, were experiencing a hospital birth. Lay midwives in the North were almost entirely of European descent and were soon surplus to requirements. Having defined midwifery to be a "relic of barbarism," American physicians actively pressed forward with the promotion of scientific childbirth, placing what had always been perceived as a fundamentally natural physiological event securely into the realm of pathology requiring medical expertise.[4] New concepts of asepsis, analgesia, and sedation during labor coincided with the professionalization of medicine, creating an atmosphere of expanding scientific horizons for the new medical specialty of obstetrics. In order to attract talented physicians to the field, clinical experience and experimentation was offered in the growing number of hospitals providing maternity care to impoverished urban women. Here, women experienced an actively managed labor consisting of heavy sedation, the elimination of the second stage of labor by the use of forceps, and the manual extraction of the placenta. Middle- and upper-class women with the luxury of choice selected a medically managed, hospital birth, too. It was perceived to be a symbol of modernity and progress and reflected the trend toward full acceptance of medical authority and knowledge.[5]

Social and cultural changes only peripherally related to childbirth solidified the shift to medicalized hospital birth. Access to mass transportation, automobile ownership, and availability of contraception all contributed to the widening embrace of modern methods and technology. A gradual diminishing of ethnic identity and the restriction on immigration led women to view physician-managed birth as a mark of distinction, figuratively connecting them to American womanhood.[6] In the mid-1920s approximately 50 percent of all births in large cities took place in hospitals, and by 1940 that figure had increased to 75 percent. However, physician-assisted hospital birth did not initially lower maternal mortality rates. In fact, the national maternal death rate in 1932 stood at 63 deaths per 10,000, up from the 1915 rate of 60 per 10,000. Significantly, the mortality rate in urban areas, where hospital birth had become commonplace, was higher than the national average. It was not until the widespread use of antibiotics in the years surrounding World War Two that maternal mortality began to decline rapidly.[7]

Comparative figures for the southern states are difficult to assess with any accuracy largely due to the incomplete, often nonexistent, records of vital statistics from the early decades of the twentieth century. Suffice it to say, the almost total neglect of the health needs of the African American population in the Jim Crow South created an indescribable level of chronic ill health, the depth of which was not fully realized until federal government physicians assessed the region in the 1960s.[8] Poor health, deficient housing and sanitation, exacerbated by an inadequate medical infrastructure and institutional discrimination had taken its toll. Lay midwife Margaret Charles Smith from Eutaw, Alabama, traveled almost two hundred miles to Tuskegee's Andrew Memorial Hospital in the event of one of her patients requiring emergency treatment; it was the closest hospital that she was confident would admit black patients.[9] As late as 1942, there were 112 hospital beds in Mississippi for a black population of one million, and the black doctor to population ratio was the worst in the country: 18,000 people for every black physician.[10] Firmly established impediments based on race restricted the number of African American doctors, and those that persevered tended to practice in towns that could sustain a black middle-class patient base. Many white doctors felt no obligation to see black patients. Some feared that by caring for black patients they would lose their white clientele as a result, or because of the real or presumed inability of a patient to pay for treatment, they preferred to not risk financial insecurity.

In this isolation, midwifery endured and the elevated position of the midwife continued in its centrality to community networks and relationships. With no opposition, midwives continued to transmit or "mother" the culture of African American womanhood, and they perpetuated the relational vision of health in their role as generational mediators. In doing so, they constructed a sense of shared heritage and cultural stability in an uncertain world; grandmothers, mothers, daughters, and granddaughters through shared experience understood the essence of what it was to be an African American woman.[11] The continuity across generations is reflected in the appellation "granny midwife." Onnie Lee Logan remembers people saying, "That yo' granny. That's yo' grannymother. She delivered you. She's the one that first put her hands on you. She's the one that made you cry, got the breath in you."[12] Children and adults often visited their "granny" midwife on birthdays or important life milestones. Delivering women across generations of a family brought joy to midwives and reinforced their sustained presence in the community. Claudine Curry Smith, a midwife in Virginia, recalled that to see a child that she delivered reach maturity, and then attend her in childbirth was one of her greatest pleasures.[13]

This sense of intergenerational female connectedness was not limited to the women they served. Particularly exhibited in the older midwives on whom there is documentation, there was a powerful matrilineal obligation to continue the vocation; midwives were the daughters, nieces, and granddaughters of midwives. Onnie Lee Logan's mother was a locally respected midwife as supervision and licensing began in the early 1920s, but she never declared herself as being active with the county health officials. However, it

was Mrs. Logan's grandmother, once an enslaved midwife, whom she credits
for the inspiration to follow in the tradition.[14] Their obligation to the role
generally overruled any reluctance they had to serving as a midwife. Louvenia
Taylor Benjamin, midwife of Baldwin County, Alabama, preferred to be a
teacher and conceded, "I just didn't want that midwife business, although my
grandmother was one and I knew I inherited it."[15] Margaret Charles Smith
was adamantly opposed to it. Her local doctor had observed her assisting
her cousin in labor, and he asked that she become a licensed midwife. She
told him in no uncertain terms, "No sir, nobody's going to turn me into a
midwife." She had no interest in staying away from home all night and having
"no coffee next morning. . . . nowhere to wash your face, and you look like
you've come out of the sewer pipe."[16] It was a commitment to her Christian
duty to people in need, instilled in her by her grandmother, that convinced
her otherwise. There was a great reverence and love for their matriarchal role
model, be it a mother, grandmother, or aunt. It was to her they looked for
strength and guidance in life. Margaret Charles Smith's relationship with her
grandmother was profound, and her reverence for her "Mama" delayed her
own marriage. This deep sense of commitment to a woman who was once
"put on a stage and sold for three dollars" and had only one child but raised
ten others, connected Mrs. Smith to the past and guided her future as she
continued to live by the example set by her matriarch.[17]

A religious calling was fundamental to the work of the midwives. Despite
traditional knowledge and skill, they relied on their spirituality to guide their
actions; in fact, prayer and spirituals were integral features of childbirth. Onnie Lee Logan described her God-given wisdom as "motherwit," and during
her many years of practice she always "kep' God in front."[18] Other midwives
claimed to have "some kind of feeling knowing they are always blessed"
or that they "take the Lord into their insides" before they act.[19] Elizabeth
Singleton, in recounting her experience, remarked, "The good Lord taught
me how to catch babies . . . when I was catching babies, I would pray for you.
I would ask the Lord to help me take care of you."[20] Onnie Lee Logan, when
faced with having to resuscitate a newborn, recalled that she "pitched out on
what God told [her] to do, and forgot about books and other people."[21] With
utmost confidence in her God-given "motherwit" and having never been
taught cardiopulmonary resuscitation, she performed gentle chest compres-
sions with artificial respiration until an unresponsive newborn cried and was
able to sustain its own respiration.[22]

Several midwives were elevated to the status of "Mother of the Church," a
revered position of spiritual wisdom at a time when spiritual leadership was

patriarchal.[23] Childbirth was recognized as a dangerous event in a woman's life and the perception of doing "God's work" necessitated an element of fatalism on the part of the midwife, the will of God being served in death as well as in life.[24] Louvenia Taylor Benjamin's words speak for all her colleagues: "Anytime, anytime I'd have a case, I would always tell the Lord before I went and then I'd thank Him afterwards, after I delivered."[25] This was just one aspect of the African American lay midwife's philosophy that was in direct opposition to the medical establishment's absolute acknowledgment of the preeminence of scientific methods.

Although some traditional treatments clearly conflicted with conventional medical wisdom, some folk practices employed by midwives were compatible with scientific theory. For example, in a 1926 monograph, *Folk beliefs of the Southern Negro*, Newbell Niles Puckett observed that "almost everywhere the linen bandage used during childbirth must be scorched before applying, a practice with some distinct sanitary advantages." Preparations containing spiderwebs, soot, and cherry tree bark, all natural coagulants, were used to treat hemorrhage.[26] By the time Onnie Lee Logan was in practice, manufactured salves and treatments were available such as Vicks, and she distanced herself from home-grown remedies, admitting relief that she was not reliant on them. However, recalling her grandmother's preparations of all sorts of herbals teas Mrs. Logan insisted that some of them worked, "Through God it [they] worked."[27]

A midwife's pivotal position in the community as a transmitter of culture, folklore, and spirituality was only one facet of her empowerment. Midwives had not the advantage of formal education and yet they had an innate resourcefulness or in Onnie Lee Logan's words, an ability to "use whatcha got."[28] Midwives saw themselves as "poor people who missed an opportunity to pursue an education," but midwifery allowed them to put their "big minds to work" and learn empirically through experience and evidence gathering.[29] Complex decision making combined with compassionate caring allowed midwives to function as autonomous, independent practitioners, and they met few problems they could not overcome with the help of their community.

A feature common to lay midwives is that their families were not quite as economically vulnerable as most in their communities. Onnie Lee Logan's father owned land, farmed, and had a carpentry business making funeral caskets for black and white customers. She said, "we never had to sharecrop for nobody . . . but we stayed humble." Her mother taught her to "stay down, stay lil, stay humble, and serve God. That's where yo' blessin's come from."[30] That is not to say that Mrs. Logan's life was not one of hard physical work and hardship; it was, but she was aware of the comparison between herself and poorer members of her community who were trapped in a desperate cycle of poverty and deprivation. Margaret Charles Smith, Claudine Curry Smith, and Gladys Milton also share stories providing evidence of their families' subtle advantage and good reputation within the community. Gladys Milton's aunt and lay midwife, Aunt Mag, was accused of "trying to be white" but always retaliated by saying, "you don't have to be rich to be clean and neat."[31] In fact, once midwifery was brought under supervision by the state the stipulations for licensing included good standing in the community and demonstrated cleanliness of person, home, and character. A white public health nurse in Georgia observed this common theme in the midwives she supervised. She said, "Of all the dozens of colored midwives I have visited I have yet to see one who did not have flowers growing somehow, somewhere, about her place." At one home, the nurse noted the visible broom marks across a large front yard![32]

Midwifery services were never withheld for lack of monetary payment, but the cash-poor clients paid what they could in all manner of ways; services were offered, produce exchanged, and promises made, but not always kept. Mary B. Hilliard's mother was a midwife in Natchez, Mississippi, before licensing began. She charged three dollars for her services but often accepted produce when need be.[33] Once assigned by the county, fees increased incrementally from five dollars to ten, then fifteen, up to twenty and even fifty dollars in Margaret Charles Smith's town of Eutaw, Alabama.[34] Anecdotes abound on the topic as midwives grumbled about nonpayment. One midwife bemoaned the fact that she accepted a bushel of cornmeal as payment only to discover that it was infested with weevils. However, another struck it lucky with her payment of a dog that eventually produced an offspring worth $600.[35]

"Lord, have mercy, if I just had the money that folks owed me" was a common cry from midwives who were themselves financially poor. Margaret Charles Smith was not averse to reminding mothers and fathers of adult children that she was never reimbursed for her services years previously. "I just give it to them. I'm short," she admitted, she needed the income.[36] Mamie Reed, a Leflore County midwife in Mississippi, went a step too far when, after several weeks of nonpayment, she took the baby she delivered as collateral, and promptly found herself under arrest for kidnapping. A county officer explained: "Perhaps this Mamie Reed had been used to buying things on the installment plan, and thought the same principle could be applied to her services."[37] Naturally, this was an exception to the rule and midwives' dreams

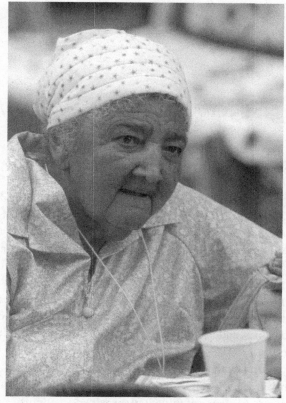

Margaret Charles Smith at the 1990 Alabama Folklife Festival in Birmingham, Alabama. Alabama Department of Archives and History.

of cash payment paled in comparison to their vocation. All grumbling and grievances aside, Claudine Curry Smith exhibited the customary principle when reassuring a sixteen-year-old without any means of payment. She told her, "Now listen, if I don't get paid for that baby, if I deliver it for you, God will pay me. I'm already paid because I got two legs and two good arms and hands."[38]

Midwifery's deeply engrained cultural motifs of spirituality, authority to practice, and matriarchy extended by necessity out of enslavement, emancipation, and beyond. As regulation and supervision began, these inherent characteristics placed lay midwives in an ideal position to conserve childbirth tradition, but yet embrace change and gently modify the culture to the advantage of the women they served.

CHAPTER 3

LICENSING AND THE "NEW LAWS"

Significant change was underway by the early 1920s. Conclusions from government studies identified three chief causes for the poor maternal mortality figures: general ignorance of the dangers associated with childbirth, the need for skilled care and proper hygiene, and poor access to adequate obstetric care.[1] In response, Progressive Era proponents for improvements in maternal and child health steered through Congress the Sheppard-Towner Maternity and Infancy Protection Act in 1921. This law provided grants to states in order for them to meet the health needs of expectant mothers and newborns, the states being required to match federal dollars. Under the mandates of the act, federal funding was made available to cover the cost of state programs for mothers and babies, and in 1922 and 1923 Alabama, for example, had a purse of over $35,000 allocated for the "provision of instruction in the hygiene of maternity and infancy through public health nursing, consultation centers, and other suitable methods."[2]

The protracted existence of midwifery provided an opportunity for poor African American women to interface with state and local government for the first time. Without an extensive health-care infrastructure, midwifery was accepted as a necessary, albeit temporary measure, and primary among the goals of state departments of health was the need to license all midwives deemed capable of training, and restrict the practice of those too elderly or unfit. In addition, the care had to be standardized and the midwives trained in rudimentary techniques of hygiene and asepsis. To lower maternal mortality two essential objectives had to be achieved: control of puerperal infection, and educate the midwives to call a physician with any deviation from normal pregnancy and labor. In Mississippi, the program was firmly described as one of supervision, not promotion, and on June 1, 1921, Mrs. Jean Reid, RN, was appointed as the first supervisor of midwives by the State Board of Health. Soon after, the responsibility fell under the purview of the Department of Public Health Nursing, and its supervisor, Mary D. Osborne, remained in the post for decades, earning the admiration of officials and lay midwives alike. After an initial survey by the Bureau of Child Welfare, Mississippi was found to have approximately 5,000 active midwives, and after assessing each woman individually 4,209 were officially recognized.[3] States across the South established midwifery control in a similar way. When Robeson County, North Carolina, initiated a midwifery program, county health officers registered 128 women, 100 were black; the average age of the group was fifty-six, and thirty-eight were literate. An eligible midwife had to be in good standing with the community and be considered of high moral repute. Her good general health was determined by a medical examination, and she had to be inoculated against typhoid fever and vaccinated against smallpox. Importantly, given the prevalence of syphilis in the South, a negative Wassermann blood test was critical to her being awarded a license to practice. Thirteen midwives in Robeson County's initial group tested positive for syphilis. Being able and willing to abide by directions set by the county health department was a requirement, and she must be seen to maintain high standards of personal and domestic hygiene.[4]

The supervisory aspect of the regulations governed the annual license renewal. To remain in good favor with the county and state, each midwife was required to firmly adhere to the "new laws" that were detailed in the midwives' manual of permitted practice. Each year she had to undertake a medical examination to ensure her physical health, and as the supervisory programs became more refined longer-term health screenings were implemented. For example, a midwife practicing in Mississippi in the 1940s had the Wassermann blood test for syphilis on even-numbered years, and a chest x-ray for tuberculosis on odd-numbered years.[5] Her regular attendance at midwife meetings was mandatory, and she was required to maintain regular contact with the board of health by submitting birth certificates in accordance with the law, and updating the county with details of any new patients she had acquired. With the supervision fully established, individual record cards were kept documenting any complaints against the midwife, all her deliveries and birth certificates on file, her willingness to follow instruction, her club and training attendance, and the results of her health screening.[6]

Despite the evident need for the continued dependence on lay midwives, some officials and physicians were doubtful that any poorly educated black woman was capable of delivering an elevated standard of care, or was even worthy of the time and energy required to achieve such a goal. In North Carolina, the medical officer of the Robeson County Health Department observed that the typical midwife in the rural South is "far below the European midwife in intelligence and no training under the sun could make

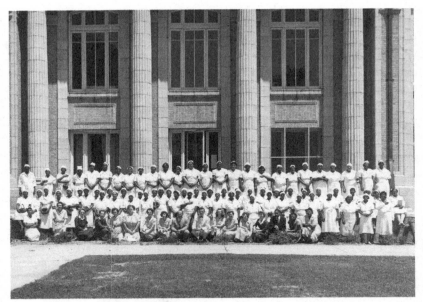

Bolivar County Midwives Meeting, 1951. Courtesy of the Archives and Records Services Division, Mississippi Department of Archives and History.

her a competent obstetric attendant."[7] Likewise, when supervision began in Mississippi, a large number of physicians believed that "very little could be done with the ignorant midwives, and not a few asserted that any attempt to change the situation would be a hopeless task."[8] In reality, this attitude was soon proven entirely wrong; the supervision of midwifery practice led to the creation of an unexpected cadre of African American health workers.[9]

From the outset, lay midwives actively engaged in the reforms launched by Sheppard-Towner. To rapidly raise the standards of care, one condition of practice was to attend a series of instructional sessions that served three purposes: to inform the midwives of the "new laws" that would govern their practice in the future, to teach techniques of asepsis and personal cleanliness, and to monitor and license compliant practitioners on an annual basis. County-based public health nurses were assigned the task of teaching small groups of midwives, and efforts were made to circumvent the limited educational attainment of the midwives, a high proportional of whom could not read or write.[10] Emphasis was placed on the invaluable service provided by the midwives, and their double responsibility to mother and baby. However, it was instilled in the midwives that because they were now integrated into the state system, only by embracing the new laws and supervision could they fulfill their commitment. This expectation on the part of the state boards of health represented a sea change for the lay midwives who until that point had been accustomed to practicing autonomously.

Department of health officials generally observed and recorded a positive response to the training from the midwives. They were eager to learn and attended the compulsory classes despite many having to travel a distance to the designated meeting places, often twenty to thirty miles. Walking was the only option for many, and to make certain she was punctual for a morning meeting, one woman's walk was long enough to require an overnight stop at a friend's home.[11] One of midwifery's harshest critics commended his county's midwives on their cooperation: of the 128 midwives in Robeson County, an average attendance of 90 was recorded for all the classes during the first five years of regulation.[12] Early in the training program offered at the Andrew Memorial Hospital in Tuskegee, Mississippi, the instructor, Dr. Kenney, observed: "It was interesting to see these women, some in their seventies, many of whom had never attended a day of school in their lives, come back and forth daily for their instruction. They were very enthusiastic over the work given them."[13] These optimistic sentiments were similar to the prediction of supervisor Lois Trabert of the Mississippi Bureau of Child Welfare when she proclaimed in 1923, "I firmly believe that when we do get these midwives properly trained, in as far as that is possible, they will do better and cleaner work than the average country doctor."[14] She was correct in her assessment; within three years Dr. Felix J. Underwood of the Mississippi State Board of Health reported extremely positive results in his evaluation of the midwifery program. In his 1925 survey of physicians he received many appreciative comments about the "splendid cooperation on the part of the midwives."[15]

In 1924, Katherine Hagquist, supervisor of midwifery control measures, was assigned the task of assessing midwives in Texas; her narrow survey addressed the situation in only fifteen counties, most in the southeast part of the state. Although initially skeptical of their ability to learn, she acknowledged that the midwives were, "almost without exception, eager to attend classes of instruction and one could see a decided change in their personal appearance after having attended a few lectures and demonstrations."[16] Across the region these early training programs were recorded a success when, like a butterfly emerging from a cocoon, the midwives were transformed from a "disorderly and dirty group of tobacco-chewing women" into a well-behaved class of pseudo-nurses wearing starched white aprons; they were cleansed of the negativity of their race and gender.[17]

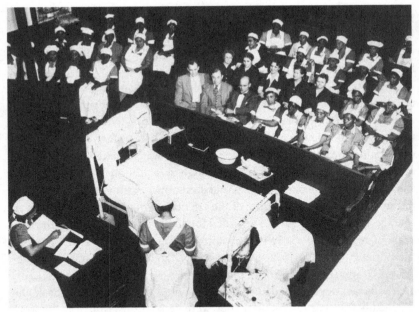

A church used as a classroom for training midwives. American College of Nurse-Midwives. American College of Nurse-Midwives Records. 1946–1978. Located in: Modern Manuscripts Collection, History of Medicine Division, National Library of Medicine, Bethesda, MD; MS C 330.

To reinforce the regulations under which the lay midwives now had to practice, monthly midwife club meetings became the primary method of ongoing supervision; in fact, Felix Underwood considered the local club meetings to be the single most effective element of the supervisory program in Mississippi. Beyond the main goal of disseminating information to midwives, the clubs connected the growing county health system to the most isolated communities. Moreover, club meetings enabled midwives to retain some control of their work and to enhance their position as community leaders while also representing the unfamiliar realm of professional health care; they were allowed to be responsible for the success of their own club. Outside of the required elements of the meeting the midwives were encouraged to initiate and plan their work in the community, which soon incorporated public health in addition to maternal health. From among the group members of preferably around ten midwives, a club leader was appointed by the public health nurse, and the group elected a club secretary, each position coming with its own set of responsibilities designated in the midwives' manual of practice. Essentially, the club leader was an extension of the public health department. Her responsibilities were largely involved with ensuring that club members were conforming to the regulations; she inspected equipment, distributed eye drops for infants, and submitted a report to the supervisor. In contrast, the secretary had a more administrative function, taking roll, keeping meeting minutes, and assisting members with the completion of birth certificates.[18]

With the leader presiding, each meeting was opened with a prayer, sometimes a specific prayer for midwives:

> Almighty God, our heavenly father, the Author and Finisher of our lives, we give thee thanks for health and strength and all the joys of life.
>
> We pray that wouldst bless the mother and fathers everywhere, make them more loving in their hearts, and more Christ-like in the things they say and do.
>
> Guide us in this meeting, and may it be the means of preparing midwives to render service more pleasing to Thee, and more acceptable to our fellow man.
>
> May Thy will be done and Thy kingdom come everywhere and when our work be done grant us that we may enter the building of God, the house not made with hands, eternal in the heavens. In Jesus' name. Amen.[19]

What followed was a familiar agenda: roll was taken, minutes read, equipment checked, and supplies distributed. The following is an excerpt from a club meeting report: "At 10 am the leader called the house to order by singing the midwife song and reading a chapter of Mark. The leader inspected the bags and they were all ok, and called the roll, three were absent, and the secretary read the minutes of the last meeting. We read the midwife manual on page 27 and 28 and talked [about] how we would arrange our meetings. We want our supervisor to see we plan to do more. We wish these meetings had started years ago."[20] When able to attend, the public health nurse was allocated ten to twenty minutes for demonstration or teaching, but she was advised against monopolizing the meeting, which was firmly the domain of the club leader. "The Midwives Song" was included in every meeting and sung with accompanying hand motions to reinforce principles of hygiene (please see chapter 7). With the clubs well established by the 1940s, one physician observer reported a meeting with a "business-like atmosphere" being presided over by an efficient midwife leader and club secretary.[21]

The clubs helped to maintain morale and also created an environment where peer pressure elevated individual performance. Having formally worked independently, this sense of teamwork and support was welcomed by most. The club meetings provided a venue for midwives to interact with public health nurses and learn to utilize them as a resource when necessary. In turn, nurses were encouraged to "know the midwives as individuals" so as foster the desired level of trust, but in their supervisory role they were advised: "Firmness is needed on occasion; understanding should be a prerequisite to its use."[22] An undercurrent of racial superiority is evident, however; in developing a greater understanding of the lay midwives, many nurses learned unexpected and profound lessons. One nurse admitted she learned "the simplicity of dignity and the dignity of simplicity."[23] Another laughingly said, "My midwives have conjured me out of my intolerance. Now I find myself staunchly defending them to doctors, to civic clubs, or any one who don't [sic] give them what I consider their dues."[24] Those who had previously thought themselves intellectually superior broadly accepted the concept of intelligence being not simply a matter of education: "The midwives who can not read or write are those who lacked the opportunity to learn, and contrary to the opinion of those not familiar with the problem, are among the best midwives. Although the rudiments of education were not available in their youth, they are nevertheless intelligent, eager for instruction, tractable, and keen in the art of observation and enlisting aid." Such was the assessment of Dr. Felix J. Underwood in 1938, after fifteen years of midwifery supervision.[25]

CHAPTER 4

IMPLEMENTING THE CHANGES

Annual Report for the Lee County Midwife Club[1]
    We, the midwives of Lee County are glad to make this report. We have through the help of God, had more success this year than ever before. We have had better attendance, better progress, more interest than ever before.
    Through the help of the white nurses, we have improved our people 100 percent. We are thankful that we have had lectures from preachers at our club meetings on midwives in a scripture way, which give all midwives a new thought, a new mind to understand the manual and get more out of it. We asked our pastors of different churches to stress our "Clean Up Campaign" and teach cleaniness [sic] through their church program. We visit sick rooms, lend a helping hand to the needy, and this year 1937, the midwives has delivered 124 babies and registered the same.
    We have all been in love and union with each other, have tried to live up to our training from the nurses, and we want to assure them that we do appreciate what they has done for us, because through the Health Department, Doctors and Nurses, we have been brought to light, and are so thankful that we try to keep this in mind.
    That we profit in proportion as we glorify and dignify our daily task, and as we put brains and skill into common occupation of life.
    We expect to do better in the year of 1938 than ever before.

Secretary of the Club,
Lillie Bell Hill

Clearly, African American lay midwives were ideally positioned to significantly raise the standard of maternity care. Their acceptance of their pivotal role in the community together with an eagerness to expand their knowledge base suggests that the midwives were well aware of the potential for

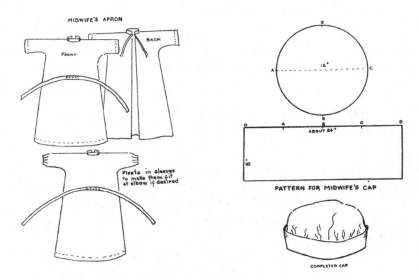

Instructions for gown and cap, Virginia Midwives Manual.

positive change. A critical component of the "new laws" was the mandate that all pregnant women required a physical examination by a physician to be approved for a midwife delivery, and accordingly midwives efficiently marshaled their clients into the nearest prenatal clinic. Midwife training classes and prenatal clinics became the nexus for combining micro and macro components of care: the clinics providing a link to medical expertise, a dimension of macro-level of health-care provision not previously available to poor women; the training classes functioning as a vehicle through which elements of scientific care could be disseminated to lay providers. Unlike the situation currently experienced by many poor rural women with limited access to prenatal care, lay midwives were plugged into the community ready and fundamentally suited to providing "hands-on, boots on the ground" micro-level maternity care.

The midwives' ability to "use whatcha got" was quickly enhanced by the science-based knowledge imparted during training sessions. While some midwives had already made the connection between maternal well-being and cleanliness, ostensibly all now adopted the dictates of the "new law" concerning hygiene, and the concept of cleanliness was stressed repeatedly. Onnie Lee Logan embraced what she called the "good rules and regulations" that substantially upgraded the standard of care: "When I go to a deliver a

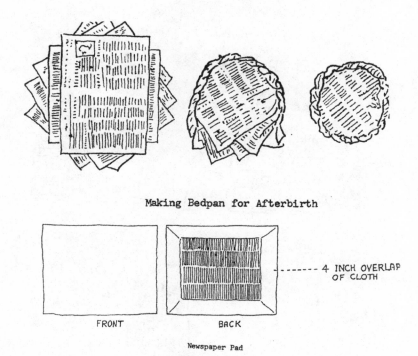

Making Bedpan for Afterbirth

FRONT BACK

4 INCH OVERLAP OF CLOTH

Newspaper Pad

Instructions for making pads and receptacles in *The Alabama Midwife: Her Book*, 1956. Alabama Department of Public Health, Montgomery, Alabama.

baby I wear all white. All white. My white coat. All white. We wears a lil white cap. That's a lil white cap comes around here tied to my head. It's mo' sanitary than havin' yo' hair loose."[2] The state departments of health provided patterns for making the caps and gowns so the midwives could equip themselves appropriately; most included them in the manual. Directions for sterilizing were explicit: cloth items such as these were to be "washed, boiled, ironed, and together wrapped in a clean white cloth three fourths of a yard square."[3]

They were receptive to ideas that provided a better environment for themselves and the women they served. Because the midwives were fully embedded in their communities they saw immediately where and how improvements could be made. In the past women delivered on quilts that the midwives later had to wash and sterilize, but after some basic instruction in class, midwives refined techniques to make disposable pads, receptacles, and sanitary towels from newspaper. The midwife's instructional manual emphasized the importance of preparation to ensure a clean environment at

LESSON IV.—MAKING THE SUPPLIES

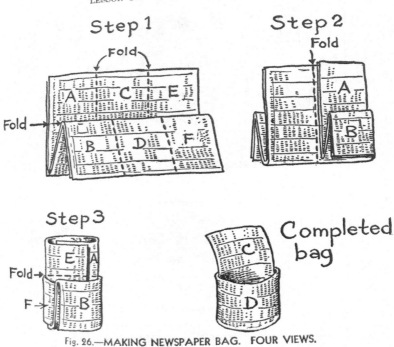

Fig. 26.—MAKING NEWSPAPER BAG.   FOUR VIEWS.

Instructions for making a newspaper bag in *Manual for Teaching Midwives*. Reynolds-Finley Historical Library, the University of Alabama at Birmingham.

delivery is maintained, and gave instruction on how to make the necessary equipment.[4]

Ideally, the midwife began preparing for delivery early in a woman's pregnancy. Aside from prenatal clinic visits, at least three home visits were recommended during pregnancy, and the manual stipulated the goals of each visit as far as a practical preparation for delivery went. A list of essential supplies was left with the mother on the first visit, and instruction on the importance of a clean home. If required the midwife taught the mother how to meet her expectations of cleanliness. During the second visit at around the seventh month of pregnancy, the midwife demonstrated how to make the necessary equipment: protective pads for the bed, waste holders, sanitary pads, cotton wool balls. It was an opportunity to get to know a mother during the pregnancy, developing a deeper, trusting relationship with her as well as ensuring that practical matters were addressed before delivery. Onnie Lee Logan explained, "[I'd] go and visit 'em. Talk with 'em. Look at the bed. See how the bed's set up cause I cain't work left-handed. You have all that in front so when you got there you didn't have to start makin' preparations for that."[5] The home visits encouraged the involvement of the baby's father, and the midwife helped him anticipate the inevitable changes as the pregnancy progressed. Preparing any older children for a newborn sibling was another important aspect of the home visits. The midwife's obligation was that the family viewed her as "a friend and helper."[6] Managing safe childbirth requires planning and supplies. Moreover, safely delivering women in isolated homes without power or proper sanitation required assistance, a person to attend to a fire, boil water, ensure the lighting is adequate, or go for help in the event of an emergency. Having the reciprocated support and trust of the family was essential.

In reality, many women went into labor having completed little preparation, and the midwives had to be adept at rapid response. They always had their delivery packs and bags clean and ready to use as per the manual, but in addition they carried with them a supply of clean sheets, newspapers, and sterile pads. The midwives were responsible for certain types of dressings, their regular equipment, and their uniform, all of which needed to be either clean or sterile per directions in the manual. The "book," as some called it, instructed them on techniques for doing so: using a hot iron to press the large pads and for storage folding them toward the center keeping the inner surface clean; placing a potato in the oven with the dressings, and once the potato was cooked the dressings were presumed to be sterile and ready to use.[7]

These tremendously important, literally lifesaving, principles of hygiene were passed on to the community one family at a time as the lay midwives engaged with each expectant woman. However, despite the fact that the Sheppard-Towner Act was repealed in 1927 under heavy opposition from the American Medical Association, innovative programs designed to enhance midwifery care continued to gain momentum. In Mississippi, Mary D. Osborne, the supervisor of Public Health Nursing, initiated a home demonstration program in late 1931, whereby each midwife was required to set up a delivery room in her home for public viewing. The campaign was doubly effective. Not only was it a community health educational opportunity, but it also provided a mechanism by which lay midwives could be annually assessed and standards of hygiene maintained. Instructions in the manual were precise. The midwife had to advertise her demonstration at least two

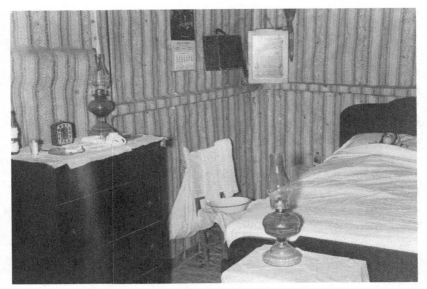

Demonstration delivery room. Courtesy of the Archives and Records Services Division, Mississippi Department of Archives and History.

weeks in advance, and she was advised to select a date "after the cotton is chopped and after it is picked" so as to attract the maximum number of visitors. A sign-in sheet for guests was made available and a brief written response to the exhibit encouraged. The room set up exactly as a delivery room enabled prospective mothers to better realize what was required of her in terms of preparation and allowed her to understand more fully the reasons for doing so. The midwives were given the opportunity to practice and "learn to do by doing."[8] The public health nurse ensured that attention was paid to every minute detail of the room, and the midwife sent a report to the department of health. In 1938, 1,165 lay midwives set up demonstration rooms, some to which as many as one hundred visitors attended. Black and white, male and female, plantation owners and tenant farmers, insurance agents and physicians viewed the room and had the opportunity to question the midwife. The demonstrations revealed to the wider community the extent to which the midwives had progressed. After his visit, one physician wrote: "This is par excellent, only more doctors should know about this and by all means more laymen." As testament to midwife Matilda Holt Mitchell's resourcefulness, one visitor was inspired by what could be accomplished with so little. The visitor observed that with few resources, "old ideas and methods have been relegated and replaced by the modern, scientific and streamlined ideas and methods." Their embeddedness in the local community enabled lay midwives to effectively teach principles of hygiene and preparedness in a nonthreatening environment. Dr. Felix Underwood acknowledged the success of the program and credited it for its role in reducing the maternal and infant mortality rate.[9]

However, the transfer of the ideal model to the real world was sometimes problematic. Each licensed midwife was required to carry with her at all times the instructional manual that dictated her scope of practice and any deviation could jeopardize her ability to practice legally. But providing maternity services in the homes of the desperately poor usually came down to inventive improvisation within the boundaries of the standards set by the board of health. In reality, despite the professed requirements of the county health department, the midwives were pragmatic enough to accept that sometimes a situation was less than optimal. Under these circumstances Margaret Charles Smith would tell herself: "Well, shit, can't nobody prepare what they don't have," and lay midwives took it upon themselves to teach women how to make do with what was available in terms of having a clean household and good personal hygiene.[10] Fortunately, Margaret Charles Smith was someone who could "make a way out of no way."[11] Onnie Lee Logan lamented the fact that poor black people had never been taught personal hygiene and she felt that "copycattin'" was the best way to proceed. Her philosophy was that once one household was neat and clean, other families would follow suit, thus explaining why the home demonstrations in Mississippi were so effective. During her early years as a midwife most of her families were desperately poor, large families living in two bedrooms and a kitchen, "no livin room. No bathroom. No nothing." After telling the mother firmly, "Unh, unh, I cain't deliver a baby in here. You gonna have to clean this up. I'm not allowed to deliver in here." She personally supervised the cleaning, gently teaching and advising.[12] As one midwife said: "Oh Lord, I had a white uniform and when I come home, I looked like I'd been up the chimney and slid down."[13] Claudine Curry Smith was quick to acknowledge that many of the poorest families were too proud to ask for help. It became common practice for the midwives to take their own sheets to a delivery if the mother was not thought able to create a clean environment in which to deliver, as well as soap, baby clothes, and food if needed.[14] In the most dire of circumstances, an old skirt or shirt was used to sew simple garments for the baby if there was sufficient time during the early stages of labor. There was nothing they would not do to ease the misery of poverty. Mrs. Curry Smith remembered the community support she experienced: "You know everybody was neighborly back then. If something happened, everybody fell right in to help you. That's what made it nice, in all my deliveries I've ever been on."[15] This familiarity with the families they served and the collective philosophy of self-help allowed the midwives to better meet the specific individual needs of the mother.

Essentially, the ultimate objective of midwife supervision was two-fold: to teach hygiene and asepsis with the intent of reducing maternal mortality from infection, and to train midwives to report abnormalities to a physician and ensure that all women see a doctor prenatally. With toxemia (eclampsia) being a leading cause of maternal death, moreover a preventable death with early detection and treatment, prenatal care "was the surest way to improve maternity mortality."[16] For the first time, with lay midwives as their advocates, poor black women began to have increased access to macro-level care. Beyond better access to care, it was in the interest of the midwife to encourage a woman to attend clinic as her license to practice could be revoked if she delivered a woman without documented authorization from a doctor. Furthermore, the permission slip also served as a written commitment from the doctor that he would support the midwife in the event of an obstetric emergency.

With midwives in attendance at the antenatal clinics, their familiar friendly faces were reassuring to the women, many of whom were suspicious and distrustful of white physicians and local government. Margaret Charles Smith worked at three local clinics for twenty-eight years, assisting the doctors and helping to allay any anxiety associated with the transition into the unfamiliar world of modern medicine. In a Georgia public health department educational film, midwife Mary Coley is seen accompanying a patient to a clinic appointment, simply offering emotional support as a female relative might.[17] Since the women they served wanted a midwife delivery, the lay midwives were able to use the maintenance of good health during pregnancy as leverage. The limited resources of most women accepted, the midwives taught women how to improve their diet, abstain from alcohol and tobacco, and rest when able in order to maintain their health throughout pregnancy. Onnie Lee Logan told her patients that "early visits to their physicians is better because there is probably a lot a work that need to be done befo' it's time to have the baby. It may take havin' to build up a lil blood. You need a lot of counselin befo' with yo' vitamens and all that. If they get their visits done early it will he'p em to have a nice no'mal delivery."[18]

In the absence of a physical clinic facility, midwives coordinated with their public health nurse and opened their homes as clinics in accordance to a physician's availability to attend. Individual midwives were commended for having made essential equipment available and organizing the patients so as to ensure the physician's time was most efficiently used. Kitchen tables were used for examination tables and when the clinic ran beyond the hours of daylight, kerosene lamps were lit to extend the clinic time. As an indication of the demand, some white women were "so desirous of this service that they asked and were of course permitted" to attend clinic in the midwives' homes.[19]

The accepted cultural authority and the consistency of their presence in the community, neither a feature associated with physician-led care, made midwives extremely influential in prenatal care and education, and they ushered thousands of women to clinics as counties began to organize maternal health. However, progress was slow. In Alabama, thirteen thousand black women attended 116 maternity clinics in 1941. This amounted to roughly one-third of all black expectant mothers, the mortality rate for whom was predictably much lower than the state average.[20] But clinic access was a persistent problem and maternal health advocates were appalled. By 1950 twenty-seven counties had yet to provide this most essential service despite Alabama consistently recording the highest maternal mortality rate in the nation.[21] It had been fifteen years since the maternal welfare committee of the state board of health commanded every county health officer to organize prenatal clinics.[22]

When viewed through a culturally appropriate lens, it is unsurprising that African American women did not see the necessity of a medical examination during pregnancy, or immediately accept childbirth as a pathological process; it was a normal part of womanhood. Women continued work, if they had work, until they went into labor. Some women only just managed to get home in time to make a pallet on the floor to deliver their own child.[23] Margaret Charles Smith delivered her second child herself, without assistance, remembering she had "the good Lord" to help her.[24] Onnie Lee Logan also reinforces the perceived normality of pregnancy and labor. She said, "Childbirth is not a sickness—God gonna take care of that. . . . I declare a woman gonna have a baby if she out there in the middle of the street. She gonna have it. All she need is somebody to wrap it up and put some clothes on it. Fact of business, she can get up and do that herself."[25] Many white nurses rejected this laissez-faire attitude toward childbirth and, applying the racist assumptions of the era, confirmed that African American mothers were essentially animal-like in nature. Black mothers' reluctance to engage a doctor was interpreted as an indifferent negligence toward their unborn child.[26]

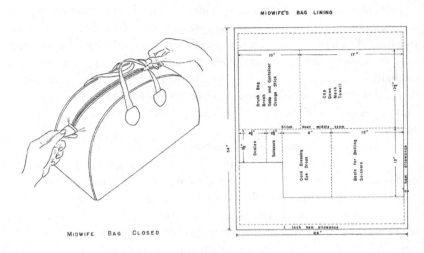

MIDWIFE'S BAG LINING

MIDWIFE BAG CLOSED

Pattern for making bag lining showing placement of permitted contents in *The Alabama Midwife: Her Book, 1956*. Alabama Department of Public Health, Montgomery, Alabama.

Beyond the perception of childbirth being a natural event, a fundamental distrust of white doctors also made black women reluctant to seek medical help even for the required prenatal examination. Again the midwife's culturally elevated position was crucial in overcoming this barrier. In her work on medical experimentation on African Americans, Harriet Washington uses the term *iatrophobia*, a fear of doctors, which she asserts, continues to detrimentally impact the health of black Americans today.[27] Onnie Lee Logan acknowledged this fear, recalling that in the past, black people were treated as less than human. She understood their hesitancy because "they thought the doctors would do some kinda experiment on 'em. Removin' this an removin' that because it was nothing but a black body."[28] Black women were afraid of being coerced into having a tubal ligation, or like the civil rights activist Fannie Lou Hamer, a hysterectomy without giving consent, a procedure referred to as a "Mississippi Appendectomy."[29] With this cultural empathy, though, the midwives were able to persuade women to undergo a medical examination during pregnancy, and provide the necessary reassurance to ensure that the women they served had access to macro-level care.

The interplay of the spiritual and psychological realms underpinned a belief in a midwife's God-given skills, and conversely a woman's confidence in the midwife was based in her acceptance that the midwife's actions were guided by a higher power. In the absence of an alternative, trust was imperative. One lady said of her midwife: "Couldn't no doctor in town or anywhere else could of made me feel any better than Mrs. Smith in assuring me that everything was going to be all right, and it was."[30]

Using this deep foundation of trust, experience, and reassurance, licensed midwives were able to distance themselves from most of the traditional treatments. In fact, the most capable midwives had removed dangerous and ineffective treatments from their repertoire prior to the enforcement of the "new laws" and state supervision. But there was no sense of disapproval of the older midwives, simply an acknowledgment that they were doing the best they could under the circumstances. Instead, Mrs. Logan placed the blame on those who neglected the poor and uneducated, leaving them with few alternatives: "I wouldn't criticize 'em [the older midwives] so much because they were doin' a job well done as fur as their knowledge would lead 'em. I don't call that ignorant." She went on, "I don't say she wasn't uncompetent. Those old Negroes in those days needed trainin'."[31] But some traditional practices such as herbal teas to augment labor, placing a knife under the bed to relieve pain, and aiding the ease of labor by having the woman wear a hat belonging to the baby's father endured despite the county health departments legislating against their use. A Virginia midwife, described by a county public health nurse as being a "brilliant" student, religiously followed her instructions on prenatal care and delivery, but held firmly to the belief that placing a pocketknife in the bed would stop after-pains.[32] However, laboring women demanded their midwives employ such methods as they brought a sense of comfort and familiarity to an anxiety-provoking experience. The placebo effect may have been responsible for the perceived efficacy and longevity of some practices. Mrs. Smith admitted that she had to stop using teas because her name became associated with "illegal" practice and she was afraid she would lose her license. Women used to ask her, "Miss Margaret, how come you are not using some of that stuff you used on Emma or Lucille? She was telling me about what good stuff you had. Why don't you give me some? Fix me some so I can get through with this baby."[33]

One method of monitoring adherence to the regulations was through bag inspections at the midwife meetings, the contents of which were non-negotiable as far as the board of health was concerned. Onnie Lee Logan recalled the midwives of her childhood having a drawstring sack containing all manner of herbs, roots, gunpowder (a clotting aid), and remedies, but licensed midwives had to follow the stipulations of the board of health. The midwife's bag was an indication of progress and responsibility. It represented a "protection for the mother and baby" against two potential killers: infection and ignorance.[34] The midwives' manual had several pages devoted to the permitted contents, and all items must be present in the bag, each having a specific place in a specially designed interior lining.[35] There was absolutely no leeway; even the external dimensions and features of the bag itself were stipulated. It had to be 14 x 6 x 10 inches, and made from "top grain cowhide with a removable lining with a clasp that stays open when the bag is open."[36] It fell to the public health nurse if in attendance or the leader of the midwives' club to oversee what some midwives called "the searching of the bag," and it was potentially stressful as is evidenced by one club's opening prayer: "Lord, we do specially ask Thee to have mercy on our head midwife who is here with us today, and who is to inspect our bags. Lord, please show her to be merciful in the inspection of those bags today!"[37] Nurses and leaders were advised to look for any sort of contraband, and in one anecdote a nurse uncovered a pistol beneath the lining of an otherwise excellent bag. The midwife admitted she was in the habit of carrying it with her on night calls and had neglected to remove it. Mortified, she pleaded, "Will you-all excuse me out of the room a minute till I get the shame off me a little?"[38] Generally, the midwives proudly kept a perfect bag that passed inspection, but some reportedly kept a bag for show and one to go!

An accurate assessment of how frequently traditional practices were used is impossible to ascertain. However, it is clear that lay midwives were often placed in a dilemma as to whether to risk possible disciplinary action or practice beyond the realm of legal stipulation. There are many documented episodes of skilled lay midwives acting beyond their formal scope of practice in the event of an emergency. Mrs. Rosie Smith from Lowndes County, Alabama, recalled delivering a woman who was bleeding as a result of a retained placenta. Mrs. Smith said, "I knew it was against the law. . . . we didn't have nobody to go get the doctor. . . . so finally I just decided. I know this is against the law, but it is against the law for you to lay there in this condition for too long." Mrs. Smith performed a manual removal of the placenta allowing the woman's uterus to contract preventing further hemorrhage. She did not lose her license, and when later praised for saving a life, she merely thanked the Lord for his guidance.[39] However, restrictions on practice gradually reinforced to both lay midwives and women that midwifery was an inadequate service that should be usurped by scientific obstetrics and that ultimate knowledge lay in the hands of doctors and the realm of macro care.

As well as their specific skills in midwifery, lay midwives also provided practical household support to the laboring women and her family. They would remain with the woman throughout labor and, in addition, often cooked and cleaned and supervised any older children. Georgia midwife Beatrice Cody asked a father of fifteen to take her to the store after delivery, and she used her $25 just earned to stock the poor family's pantry; she returned to the home and cooked them chicken and rice.[40] Onnie Lee Logan recalled that some mothers had nothing for their baby to wear and "in between contractions [she'd] take an old skirt and make somethin' for that baby to put on when it got here." Other midwives did the same.[41] This personalized care could not be replicated in the professionalized physician-led model of care. In fact, the attention to the personal, individual needs of a woman was interpreted as a sign of primitive care. Rigid order and procedure were valued more highly than flexibility and adaptability to specific needs.[42]

The midwives' official duty only required them to complete and submit a birth certificate within seven or ten days of delivery so much of their postpartum work was done on their own initiative. Some women remember midwives actually staying with the mother for two weeks, cleaning, cooking, and attending to any older children, but most just returned regularly to monitor the mother and infant. Claudine Curry Smith visited "for three days straight, to check the cord." She explained, "The baby was the main reason I was coming back, but I would check the mother too. I'd ask her if everything was all right and if she didn't give me a good answer, I'd recommend her to go to the doctor. Then I'd go every other day until the cord dropped off and was all healed. Then my work was complete."[43] Mrs. Wilson, a lay midwife in Florida, used the postnatal visits to teach young mothers how to sew; the amount of attention given was dependent on the needs of the family.[44] Louvenia Taylor Benjamin recalled assuming responsibility for premature twins when the local doctor refused to see them: "I took those babies home and built a little nest for them. I put one in one end of the crib and one in the other." She commandeered the help of her elderly neighbor and between them they attended to the intensive needs of preterm twins; the babies survived and grew into "fine children."[45] In ultimate postpartum service, it was not uncommon for midwives to adopt a "gift child," an unrelated child whom they took in because of abandonment or homelessness.[46] Midwives were mothers, aunts, grannies to *all* children.

CHAPTER 5

WORKING WITH THE STATE

Carlisle, Mississippi
October 5, 1939

My dear Miss Jones,

This is to inform you that Alleen Cambell of Rocky Springs, Miss. gave birth to a baby Oct 3, 1939, weighing 7 1/4 pounds. Miss Jones while I was on this case a woman about 42 years of age came to the house where I was and she has sores all on her arms, legs, and she says she has them on her buttocks too. So I had to tell her in a nice way we could not have her around the patient, nor the baby, and to please don't come back until I could see what could be done for her. She proclaims that the family across the road from her, has the same things on them and says that is how she became infected. Now could you go out there at once to see about this. I made a lecture on the 4th Sunday in August at a church in Willows, Miss. to the people about their health also about setting up a delivery room. I advised them if they had any sores or the least suspicion they were infected with that dreaded disease syphilis to please tell someone before it is too late. So she says she heard me talk that day and when she heard I was in the neighborhood she came to tell me about it. So I advised her to stay at home until I talked with you. So if you could go out there one day I could go to their homes with you. I mean come to my home. Of course I am going to see about my baby Saturday after the Club meets. Now some of her sores are open and running, some are dry white scabs.

Estelle W. Christian, Midwife.

Miss Osborne: This is from one of the midwives who is doing so much to educate her people that I feel real proud of her and wanted you to see this letter. The woman with the "sores" has been referred to her family physician and if Wassermann test is found positive will be given treatment.

Viola M. Jones, R.N.
County Nurse[1]

An important reward of the micro-level lay midwifery system spread beyond safely delivering healthy babies. The midwives' role in the promotion of public health cannot be overstated, and they effectively became representatives of the state boards of health. Their ability to connect public health nurses with sick or disabled children or to identify and refer those suffering from tuberculosis or venereal disease quickly became irreplaceable.[2] Without this local infiltration, the sick and contagious remained out of reach of the limited state and county assistance. Midwives, eager to improve the welfare of their communities, were granted the autonomy to develop programs of their own through the local midwife clubs. Lillie Bell Hill, of the Lee County Midwives Club, describes an excellent example of this type of outreach when her midwives coordinated with local church leaders to promote their "Clean Up Campaign." Other efforts involving teachers and May Day health education programs all extended the reach of the public health departments. Following a presentation on dental health one club publicized the benefits of oral hygiene so effectively that the itinerant salesman questioned what had prompted the demand for toothpaste![3]

Midwives also partnered with the boards of health in state surveys. In Mississippi, they assisted with assessment of the blind population, and in calculating the number of disabled people for the Vocational Bureau of the Department of Education. However, midwives particularly excelled in encouraging African Americans to be vaccinated against smallpox, diphtheria, and typhoid fever. Dr. H. C. Hicks of the Bureau of Communicable Disease expressed his appreciation:

Mississippi as with other southern states was due for a rise in the incidence of typhoid fever in 1930. There was however a reduction in cases instead. It is believed that the midwives played no small part in holding down the typhoid fever rate, due to the fact that through the efforts of the midwives as urged by the leaders of the midwives clubs thousands of the colored race were inoculated against typhoid fever.

One midwife leader brought three hundred, another two hundred, to these conferences, instigated by a letter sent out by the supervisor of midwives at the request of a local health officer. The midwives played no small part in the diphtheria control program as they have consistently, where inoculation was available, influenced colored parents to bring infants and preschool children to the conferences to be protected against diphtheria.[4]

An important aspect of the midwives' public health work was their role in the prevention of blindness. The widespread prevalence of the sexually transmitted diseases gonorrhea and chlamydia forced state boards of health to actively combat ophthalmia neonatorum, and midwives were the vanguards of this effort. Each infant was treated with two drops of 1 percent silver nitrate solution to each eye at birth using the precise technique described in the manual. It was one of the few legally enforced requirements to a midwife's practice. Instituted a decade prior to midwifery supervision, the penalty for failure to administer silver nitrate drops at birth was arrest or imprisonment, but clearly, without the consistent monitoring of midwives' practice this law was almost impossible to enforce.

Calculated or not, one positive consequence of administering maternity care locally was the competition and rivalry that emerged between midwife clubs and counties. Felix Underwood noted it in his early assessment of the clubs; he observed a desire to excel that fostered a sense of teamwork, and those unable or unwilling to adapt to the new requirements were forced out of practice. Midwives were congratulated on exhibiting their home demonstrations to record-breaking numbers of viewers, or achieving the highest vaccination rates, and county public health nurses bragged about the accomplishments of "their" midwives. Vying for "Best in State" recognition is evident in correspondence to state boards of health from public health nurses, in club reports, and in home demonstration reports. This sense of competitiveness was forged via songs sung at meetings and classes. The "Song of the Midwives" urges them to fulfill their commitment to the state by working in absolute accordance to its policy, and by doing so they would ensure that their county was renowned for the modern standards of its midwives.

Conversely, midwives ensured that the fledgling health system met its obligation to the community. When she came across cases of extreme poverty, Mrs. Logan quickly reported the emergency to the board of health. She would also have no hesitation in reporting negligent or abusive parenting

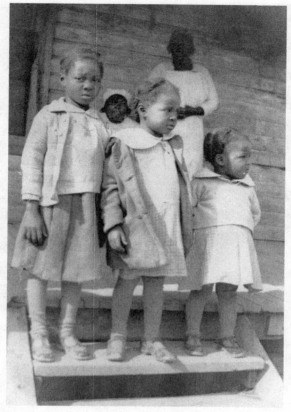

Brought by midwives for protection against smallpox, diphtheria, typhoid fever. Courtesy of the Archives and Records Services Division, Mississippi Department of Archives and History.

if she suspected it to be the case; she did a "whole lot a ministering to those broken homes."[5] Her willingness to access county services to the fullest extent on behalf of her patients is evidence of her high regard for the inclusion of midwifery as part of a legitimate branch of a multitiered health-care system. When reporting a family at risk, she was adamant that social services intervened appropriately. If a welfare agent was reluctant to take a new case on the grounds of having no evidence, Logan would respond, "All you gotta do is get up outa that office chair and investigate and you'd have yo' proof. Go by there on Friday evenin' or Saturday evenin' and see how much dope there's been and how much whiskey there's bein bought and you'd have yo' proof."[6]

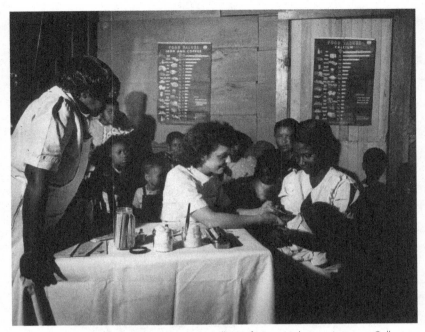

Immunizations at a midwife's home. American College of Nurse-Midwives. American College
of Nurse-Midwives Records. 1946–1978. Located in: Modern Manuscripts Collection, History
of Medicine Division, National Library of Medicine, Bethesda, MD; MS C 330.

Beyond the physical care of the woman and infant, lay midwives had a less
obvious, but essential responsibility as regards the state, that of registering
the birth, or death. Moreover, in order to make inroads into lowering a state's
maternal and infant mortality rates, an accurate and consistent method of
determining the cause of death had to be implemented. A report of Alabama's
mortality rate for 1927–1928 conclusively showed that although many deaths
were preventable, an estimated five thousand births and over fifteen hundred
deaths went unreported each year. The medical association's committee on
maternal health searched for a solution for the data collection problem, and
annually presented a critical analysis of each maternal death where statistics
allowed. It was impossible to improve care without first having an indication
of the major causes of death, and monitoring the associated trends was the
only sign of progress achieved. Despite the barrage of criticism directed
toward midwives they were tasked with a critical responsibility. However, the
data relieved lay midwives of some culpability for poor care as in 1937 physicians were in attendance in 211 of the 289 maternal deaths. In the defense
of doctors, clearly some deaths occurred during abnormal deliveries that

required medical intervention but nonetheless the committee concluded: "For every effect there must be a cause. In this instance the effect is maternal deaths; the cause, the doctors."[7]

It is perhaps surprising that the Bureau of Vital Statistics relied so heavily on midwives to collect such pivotal data, and Gertrude Jacinta Fraser explores the question in her study of midwifery in Virginia. More than facilitating a better understanding of mortality rates, the data readily exposed the degree of illegitimacy and miscegenation. Fraser argues that issues of illegitimacy, paternity, and the assignment of a racial category as part of Virginia's racial integrity laws became a wedge between midwives and women, and especially problematic was the delivery of a mixed-race child. In the event of a white woman delivering a mixed-race child, the midwife was charged with making certain that no child of a black man could ever "pass" as white, and she was compelled to assign the child a nonwhite status. According to law, the white woman must have conceived by rape, thus in registering the infant as having a black father, the midwife was in effect reinforcing the white perception of African American males being sexually aggressive. Virginia midwives were in a catch-22 situation.[8]

With the collection of accurate data imperative, all midwives' manuals had a section devoted to the proper completion and submission of state records; some directions were more explicit than others. In Alabama, the manual simply underscored the importance of filing the completed certificate with the county registrar within five days, and compelled lay midwives to enter the information clearly and accurately using "permanent ink—black, blue or blue-black." The Virginia midwives' manual listed the filing of the birth certificate as one of four legal requirements of a midwife. In a brief paragraph it warned of a fine of up to ten dollars for neglecting to register a birth. However, in South Carolina the manual provided instructions and examples for each required line item: "Item 3 Write 'Male' or 'Female.' The initial 'M' may be used for male and the initial 'F' for female."[9] To some midwives the necessity for such accurate documentation may have seemed vague and of little consequence, but a federal government teaching aid astutely reversed the beneficiaries of having accurate birth records. The emphasis was shifted away from the state and statistics toward the individual; a birth certificate being a passport to life allowing a person to begin school, to acquire a driving license, to vote, to marry, to join the military, or to receive a retirement pension.[10] Nurse-midwife Eugenia Broughton composed a song that focused on the positive benefits to the child. The lyrics of the "Birth Certificate Song" spoke of full participation in America's social, political, and economic life.[11]

Whenever you deliver perhaps a baby boy
Remember he is human, not just a little toy
His birth should be recorded within ten days or less
And in years to come you will be blessed.

We know that it's important, a solid standard rule
He'll need birth registration to enter any school
To proves he's the right age to marry or to vote
So be sure his birth date you report.

He'll need it for enlistment or maybe go abroad
Producing his birth record will prove he's not a fraud
It'll make him mighty happy if he can really say
"I'm a native of the U.S.A."

He'll then be eligible to earn an honest wage
Receive a monthly pension if he can prove his age
When sixty-five or older, he then will in due time
Live in comfort, peace and sweet sublime.

(Chorus)
Be sure his name, the date, the place are right
If not, in time he'll be in quite a plight
Check and recheck, then have the mother sign
And you will have great peace of mind.[12]

CHAPTER 6

WORKING WITH PHYSICIANS

Clearly African American lay midwives fulfilled the micro components of care that health-care policy experts believe should be integral, but are most often lacking, in care models today. However, their limited access to medical expertise and facilities at the macro level resulted in an unbalanced care that was far from optimum. Although evidence reveals many instances of mutual respect between individual lay midwives and white doctors, the midwives on whom documentation exists all decry the lack of support by the larger medical establishment. Onnie Lee Logan did not recall "a single doctor deliverin' a black baby at home."[1] Fortunately for childbearing women, lay midwives were generally confident enough in their ability and authority to demand emergency support when necessary.

Their confidence, however, met with dual problems, the scarcity of doctors across the rural South, and the inaccessibility of hospitals, both accepted as a matter of fact by the black community. The midwives determined that a more effective solution to a complication at delivery was to transfer a woman to the doctor, rather than expecting the doctor to come to the home. This strategy enabled the midwife to retain control of the situation, thereby forcing access to macro-level care. Margaret Charles Smith remembered four or five instances when she had to transport women a distance of 170 miles to Tuskegee to receive emergency care. She knew that it was in the best interest of the women to make the long journey there than to seek help at a closer hospital from which she was certain she would be turned away.[2] Claudine Curry Smith had a 70-mile drive to Richmond in the event of an obstetric emergency.[3] In describing incidents such as these, both midwives recall being stopped by the police for exceeding the speed limit. In some cases, they were able to negotiate a high-speed escort to hospital such was their reputation and authority.[4]

These recollections show the reluctance on the part of some doctors to serve poor black women, as Louvenia Taylor Benjamin experienced with the premature twins. When Gladys Milton asked if a doctor would deliver black babies, he replied, "Not if I can help it," but later did offer his services.[5] Midwifery licensing laws ensured that women received medical approval for a midwife delivery at home. Moreover, the permit committed the doctor to provide support in the event of complications. But as Claudine Curry Smith recalled, tenacity was often required to gain support from a recalcitrant doctor:

> Some [women] would come at the last minute but they had to have the card or else I couldn't deliver them. Now some of 'em would call me and hadn't been to a doctor, and I couldn't go unless I called the doctor.
>
> I called him and he said, "Well you can go up there an deliver her if you want to." Says, "she'll be all right." I said, "Dr._____, if I get up there and I need you, are you coming?" He said, "Oh she's all right," this, that and the other. I said, "Well unless you tell me you're coming I'm not going." So finally he said, "well, go ahead, but I don't think you have no problem." I said, "But you said if I have a problem you'll come. Is that what you're saying?" and he told me, "Yeah."[6]

Signs and symptoms of impending danger to mother and baby were listed in the manual, and the midwife was mandated by law to request medical assistance (for example, in cases of pre-eclampsia, seizures, hemorrhage, breech presentation, obstructed labor, et cetera). When a doctor responded to a call for help at a woman's home, the midwife ensured he met his professional and legal obligations as best she could. Maude Bryant in North Carolina summoned a doctor during an unusually difficult labor. After a cursory examination the doctor declared nothing to be wrong and prepared to leave. The midwife angrily followed him outside and firmly explained her concerns. She commanded: "Something must be done, and I want you to go back in there." She persuaded the doctor to reexamine the woman, after which he took her to a hospital.[7] Similarly, Onnie Lee Logan felt obligated to challenge an intoxicated doctor who called her an "incompetent nigra woman" after becoming belligerent and abusive; she lodged a formal complaint with the department of health.[8]

Lay midwives must be admired for their self-belief and perseverance. Although collectively the medical profession always considered midwifery to be problematic but necessary, there is much documented evidence of physicians granting lay midwives the respect they deserved. Dr. Felix Underwood, who spearheaded maternal health improvements in Mississippi, initially determined midwives to be "untrained, unlettered, and fettered by the grossest superstition," but he was quick to express his appreciation of their cooperation and to promote their accomplishments once supervision had begun.[9] In a physician survey he conducted in 1925, he reported that more than 80 percent of respondents agreed that midwives paid more attention to cleanliness (of self and equipment), and were consistently calling for medical help when necessary.[10] These were both identified as the primary goals at the onset of midwife education.

While midwifery was still considered a challenge to physicians, county boards of health, and public health nurses, it was recognized by many that midwives "did a good job where she was [they were] sorely needed."[11] Furthermore, there was encouragement from doctors for continued supervision in constructive feedback: "Urge all physicians to take an interest in their [the midwives'] work." "I note quite an improvement in the homes and attribute it to the teaching of midwives." "Education, propaganda, perseverance, keep up the good work begun." "As near as possible require higher educational standards." "No criticisms to date, puerperal trouble less, everything looks good."[12]

However, it is personal anecdotes that best represent the mutual respect between physician and midwife. Dr. Ruker Staggers worked with Margaret Charles Smith for many years and had a high regard for her ability. Local physicians trusted her decision making and knew that "if Margaret needed us [local doctors] . . . there was something going on that needed some help."[13] Likewise, Dr. Melvin Lamberth in Lower Northern Neck, Virginia, was complimentary about Claudine Curry Smith's skills, admitting that although he "taught her a few things about medicine and obstetrics, she [Claudine] taught me [him] a few things too, like how to treat people at home." He said they had a "fine relationship," and on his death in 2000, Lamberth's widow confided in Mrs. Smith and told her, "He always said you were like brother and sister."[14] It was a remarkable statement given the time and place of the friendship. Louvenia Taylor Benjamin, whom the older doctors affectionately called Professor, did not have a problem with her regular physician, Dr. Hale. He always made himself available and, if he could not go to the patient, Benjamin said he advised her by telephone when possible. She eventually earned the respect of the doctor who had refused to care for the premature twins. She explained, "He wouldn't speak to me for a long time cause I told him I didn't give a damn if he didn't do nothing [about the babies]." In town some time later, she heard a man greet her using the name Professor, and after a polite exchange about the weather, she said they became best friends: "I could go to him right now if my doctor is out of town and he'll do what he can for me."[15] The medical establishment's collective objection to midwifery was buttressed by the pervasive and derogatory gender and racial assumptions, but on an individual level the lay midwives' dedication, skill, and self-worth garnered them respect from the physicians with whom they interacted.

The cumulative effect of the advocacy of lay midwives was greater access to macro-level health care, and a standardization of midwifery care that better served women. However, the scanty distribution of physicians and hospitals across the rural South was an impediment to real improvement, and it was beyond the realm of midwives to rectify the problem. Nonetheless, even as purveyors of traditional maternity culture, under the regulations of the "new laws" lay midwives were able to adapt to and accommodate modern innovation and change for the greater good. Ultimately, though, approaching maternity care from a micro/macro perspective exposes the defects of the model. The midwives knew where their strengths and deficiencies lay, and perhaps by embracing modern change they inadvertently facilitated a more significant cultural shift that was out of their control. From their perspective, given the timelessness of midwifery, a firm assurance in their enhanced skills, and a conviction to serve, it was inconceivable that they would eventually be prohibited from practicing. Moreover, they did not foresee a time when black women would no longer seek their expertise.

PART 2

ASAFETIDA TO AUREOMYCIN

African American Nurse-Midwives

. . . probably the greatest person I have ever been privileged to know, combining a marvelous wisdom and compassion, a strength of true humility and true pride, all given direction through knowledge and purpose in a sheerly beautiful balance.

W. EUGENE SMITH ON MAUDE CALLEN, CERTIFIED NURSE-MIDWIFE

The Nurse-midwife enjoys one of the most satisfying careers in public health nursing. She sees the direct results of her work in improved health of both mothers and infants. Her visits to the home before, during and after the baby's birth frequently mean the difference between good care and poor care—or even no care at all, for each year less than a third of our Negro babies are born in hospital and many thousands of mothers go through childbirth without the care of a physician.

INTRODUCTORY STATEMENT,
TUSKEGEE SCHOOL OF NURSE-MIDWIFERY, 1945

The December 10, 1951, issue of *Life* magazine included a remarkable photo-essay that prompted an overwhelming response from its readership. It was the work of renowned photojournalist W. Eugene Smith entitled "Nurse Midwife: Maude Callen Eases the Pain of Birth, Life, and Death." The subject of the article, Maude Callen, was an African American nurse-midwife who provided vital lifesaving services to the impoverished, rural population of Berkeley County, South Carolina.[1] During the weeks following its publication, hundreds of letters and monetary donations poured in from readers, such was the overwhelming support of Mrs. Callen's selfless devotion to her community—so many donations, in fact, that she was able to establish a clinic for her patients. As a registered nurse as well as

a midwife she was described in the article as being as far removed from a
"granny" or lay midwife as "aureomycin is from asafetida."[2] In other words,
she embraced the scientific advances of modern medicine (aureomycin, an
antibiotic) and had turned her back fully on traditional, herbal remedies
(asafetida). A nurse-midwife, the article suggested, was the antithesis of a
"granny"; she was a college-educated, professional woman who embraced a
modern and scientific approach to health care.

And yet Maude Callen and her colleagues also recognized the value in
much of the care administered by lay midwives. Nurse-midwives, black and
white, provided a bridge between communities devoid of medical professionals and state and federal health-care systems. They provided a framework
under which licensed lay midwives could safely and effectively practice,
and they, like the women they supervised, were entirely committed to the
communities they served. The analogy used by Smith in his photo-essay is
indicative of the acknowledged acceptance of the march of scientific progress
during the mid-twentieth century. But those assumptions are belied by the
experience of nurse-midwives. Although a scientific approach awarded little
value to what was considered archaic, some remedies were effective and
reassuringly familiar to the community.

During the 1940s, nurse-midwives in the South found balance between
science and cultural tradition and were able to significantly improve the
childbearing experience of women there; they offered an alternative to patriarchal medical care. Working as part of a team, the nurse-midwife was
able to address both the micro and macro components of good maternal
care. She was able to compromise when necessary to adapt to the personal,
cultural, and social needs of women, and yet she was a skilled, autonomous,
professional practitioner with access, when geographically available, to the
larger medical community; she had, if you will, a foot in both camps. In
many respects nurse-midwives performed a similar role to public health
nurses; however, in contrast to nurses, all midwives share a fundamental
belief that pregnancy and birth in healthy women should be allowed to
progress naturally until it deviates from normal. Nurse-midwives were invested in midwifery as a profession, although not in traditional midwifery.
At a place and time when lay midwives were the sole providers of maternal
care for many women, nurse-midwives did not tolerate harmful superstition,
but rather coaxed, supervised, and trained capable lay midwives ushering in
a more modern maternity care.

But that balancing act came at a price. Nurse-midwifery, by its inclusion
and acknowledgment of the nonscientific aspects of care, became vulnerable

to attack by its opponents. Throughout its history in America, the profession has been plagued by challenges to its legitimacy, its professionalism, and its relevance. African American nurse-midwives faced still further impediments to practice. Given that her professional role brought her into contact with local and state governmental bodies, the macro components of care, she faced the prevalent negative forces of racial prejudice head-on, in addition to gender and professional discrimination. Whereas lay midwives were afforded some protection by their immersion at the micro, grassroots level, African American nurse-midwives were fully exposed to the debilitating constraints of working in the wider society of the Jim Crow South. Nonetheless, they were exemplars of a new approach that embraced safer, scientific care while simultaneously acknowledging the place of culture and heritage; by twenty-first century standards they were thoroughly modern practitioners, and ahead of their time.

ESTABLISHING THE PROFESSIONAL NURSE-MIDWIFE

As professionals, nurse-midwives have fought for space in a multidisciplinary arena. The origin of the struggle lies in the medical establishment's claim that embracing midwifery as a branch of nursing would lessen the prestige of obstetrics as a medical specialty, as well as create a competitive economic market for doctors. Coinciding with the period of professionalization of physicians and specialization within that group, the debate on midwifery in the early decades of the twentieth century was fervent. Obstetrician Joseph B. De Lee declared in 1915 that even a trained midwife "is a drag on the progress of the science and the art of obstetrics. Her existence stunts the one and degrades the other. For many centuries she prevented obstetrics from obtaining any standing at all among the sciences of medicine."[1] Dr. De Lee succeeded in leading the charge toward the medicalization of childbirth and from his perspective, in keeping with the promise of the scientific age, "childbirth [was] lifted out of the realm of darkness into the spotlight of new science."[2] Though this chapter argues against most of his premises, there is no denying that De Lee was an advocate for improving maternity care. He took "second place to no man or woman in [his] regard for the poor, the ignorant, the foreign-born, childbearing mother."[3] To this end he established the Chicago Maternity Center to serve the poor, immigrant community on the south side of the city. There, he and his team of physicians, medical students, and nurses provided prenatal care and free home delivery to those women previously registered with the center.

There is irony in the fact that Dr. De Lee's goals, and in many respects his actions, actually expanded the role of nurse-midwives. In 1918, a small group of mothers, obstetricians, and nurses established the Maternity Center Association (MCA) in New York City, following in the footsteps of De Lee's Chicago Maternity Center. The association set itself three tasks: to open neighborhood maternity centers in cooperation with other health agencies in the city; to find pregnant women and encourage them to use their local center for pre- and post-natal care as well as for delivery; and to study and standardize maternity care throughout the city, supported by obstetrical care.[4] It soon became apparent that few nurses were adequately equipped to provide the very specialized type of care required by a woman in childbirth.

Along with the Progressive-Era push to improve immigrant maternal care, another influence on the expansion of nurse-midwives in the United States was the contrasting path of the development of obstetric care in Europe. Unlike the situation in the United States, obstetricians in Europe felt neither competition nor animosity toward well-trained midwives practicing within a medically supervised model of care. In fact, the British parliament sanctioned the practice of midwifery in 1902 by establishing the Central Midwives Board that regulated training, conducted examinations, and certified successful candidates. The physicians on the medical board of the MCA, seeing the potential of such a system, supported a shift toward medically supervised midwifery in America. Board member Dr. Benjamin P. Watson, professor of obstetrics and gynecology at the College of Physicians and Surgeons, Colombia University, believed that "the maternal mortality in this and every other country would be materially reduced if the practice of obstetrics were in the hands of thoroughly trained midwives working in conjunction with and under the direction of properly trained doctors."[5] The editor of the *American Journal of Obstetrics and Gynecology*, Dr. George W. Kosmak, also argued for a European-style midwifery service, declaring that "there is no branch of medicine in which the nurse participates to such an important degree as in obstetrics."[6]

Although most physicians voiced their outright opposition to midwifery, or at best a grudging acceptance of midwives being a temporary but "necessary evil," some held firm as proponents of a well-trained body of midwives and of the superior service it could provide.[7] Most supporters of raising the status of midwifery and/or grafting it onto nursing were doctors who viewed the situation from a wider perspective. These allies came from the realm of public health or pediatrics and understood the role of the midwife to be greater than simply delivering a child; they recognized the value of micro factors as being essential for good maternity care. The role of the midwife, they argued, was quite different to that of the obstetrician and, to alleviate fears of economic competition, claimed that it should not "invade the province of the physician." Writing in a 1914 public health journal, Carolyn Conant Van Blarcom, a nurse educator with extensive knowledge of European midwifery regulatory programs, argued that greater value should be given to the services provided by trained midwives such as intelligent nursing care for the mother and infant during the twelve to fourteen days after delivery, advising the mother on questions of hygiene before and after delivery, as well as teaching the mother proper infant care, all services that fell outside the scope of medical practice.[8] Eminent pediatrician Dr. Abraham Jacobi, during his tenure as president of the American Medical Association in 1912, also supported a European-style midwifery service, and saw the extended role of trained midwives as an essential component of a modern, effective response to high infant mortality rates. He remarked, "A town without an ample supply of good doctors and midwives and a village without one or two competent and responsible and licensed midwives, are like a tenement house without a fire-escape or a Titanic without life-boats!"[9]

Perhaps because these ideas were new and still controversial, in New York the MCA struggled to establish a school of nurse-midwifery throughout the 1920s. Some of the most vociferous opposition came from nursing leaders themselves. They argued that public health nurses did not want to assume the added responsibility of midwifery. They, like most physicians, understood the role of the midwife in its narrowest form, a presence at birth, and underestimated the importance of thorough prenatal, postnatal, and infant care in a more holistic approach. Nurse leaders from urban public health and rural backgrounds argued that most competent nurses would be adequately prepared to manage an emergency delivery, but they were generally too busy to assume any further duties with or without additional training. Other drawbacks to nurses becoming midwives were objections to living in isolated communities where their skills were most in need, and their unwillingness to provide services for the small fee demanded by midwives. Moreover, they were afraid of tainting the reputation of public health nurses by an association with midwifery, an occupation that was disparaged by racial and class prejudice, and deemed to be unprofessional.[10]

However, by 1932 the MCA, licensed by the New York City Board of Health with supervision by the health department's Bureau of Maternal and Child Hygiene, had amalgamated with the Lobenstine Midwifery Clinic and opened as a school of nurse-midwifery, graduating its first class in 1933.[11] The governing body of MCA was pragmatic in its approach to the training of American nurse-midwives. Although they looked to Britain as a model, American needs were unique, and the goals, curriculum, and candidate requirements were modified as necessary. The initial objective of the school was to "prepare nurse-midwives to assume responsibility for the supervision, care, and instruction of women during pregnancy, labor, and the puerperium, under the guidance of a competent obstetrician."[12] Given the heavy distribution of traditional lay midwives in rural areas, particularly in the South where few physicians practiced, the school leadership recognized that in order to be successful they needed to train nurse-midwives to primarily supervise lay midwives, and to secondarily provide professional maternity care.[13] This shift in objective can be seen in the selection of students for admission. Although officially requiring that applicants be eligible for admission to university, they often overlooked this stipulation in favor of seasoned professionals, or public health nurses who were to return to areas of the country, and in fact the world, with particularly poor maternal care.[14] The dispersion of those nurse-midwives graduating between 1933 and 1953 as listed in the report published by MCA in 1953 reveals their focus on students willing to return to places of need. The success of the program lay in the blended emphasis on nurse-midwives being educators, organizers, and administrators as well as ensuring that a woman not only received safe maternity care, but also a type of care that paid attention to the social and emotional aspects of childbearing.[15]

The twenty-year report of the MCA published in 1955 applauds the successes of the program. It indicated that mortality and morbidity statistics were markedly reduced and also appraised the inclusion of the micro components of care. The report noted that the easily accessible clinic was regularly attended during pregnancy, with each woman making an average of 7.7 prenatal visits.[16] Although lay midwives were effective in steering women to clinic, they lacked the authority to control the interaction between patient and professional. Nurse-midwives accomplished both objectives. They fostered a relationship of trust creating an environment that was more conducive to counseling and education, and the women were encouraged to visit the clinic at their convenience, when they had ample time to ask questions. Moreover, anecdotes attest to how the staff made each patient feel comfortable and realize that they were genuinely interested in her welfare. The friendly atmosphere contrasted sharply to typical prenatal clinics where they found:

> Long lines of patients waiting to be seen by the physician; inadequate pre-natal care according to acceptable standards; little or no counseling of the patient; little attention paid to maternal nutrition, and little or no privacy afforded the patient or other satisfying experience, that would tend to induce the pregnant woman to register early for her antepartum care and to continue it without interruption during her pregnancy.[17]

The importance of this relationship building, MCA argued, was reflected in the fact that despite prevalent economic deprivation within the patient group, five out of six women found time to return to the clinic for a postnatal visit six weeks after delivery.[18]

The nurse-midwives graduated with a clear sense of the centrality of micro factors to good maternal care: support networks, outreach, the dissemination of knowledge in terms relevant to women, cultural perspectives. They carried this philosophy with them into their postgraduate positions; however, there were few opportunities to practice clinical nurse-midwifery. Most nurse-midwives in the 1940s and 1950s were employed as supervisors or consultants in hospitals and health departments in an extension of their public health capacities, many holding upper-level positions in public health administration.[19] Those who practiced midwifery were employed in the few federally funded demonstration projects where they conducted home deliveries, supervised and educated lay midwives, ran maternity clinics, and acted as liaisons with local health departments.

Nowhere was in greater need of their assistance than the poor, rural communities of the South, and yet the inclusion of a nurse-midwifery service into the state boards of health was entirely dependent on the senior medical officials' general perception of the midwife. Thus, the reception encountered by the New York–educated nurse-midwives varied. In 1941, the associate director of Georgia's Division of Maternal and Child Health, Edwin R. Watson, held the view that African American lay midwives' "false beliefs are fixed ideas and cannot be changed" and so was unwilling to invest in supervision and training to improve their skills.[20] However, in other southern states, medical officials claimed the atrocious maternal mortality and morbidity was as much a result of impoverished mothers having no prenatal care, often suffering from chronic disease and malnutrition, than as a consequence of care delivered by traditional midwives.[21] Dr. Hilla Sheriff of South Carolina, Dr. Frances Catherine Rothert of Arkansas, and Dr. J. N. Baker of Alabama each saw the potential benefits in the adoption of a nurse-midwifery service. In Maryland, Dr. Charles H. Peckham had his foresight confirmed when in 1939, just three years after introducing a supervising nurse-midwifery service, he declared, "In communities where a nurse-midwife has been employed the general level of obstetric care has always improved with remarkable celerity."[22]

The impressive attendance rates that the MCA earned at their prenatal clinics was in itself responsible in part for reducing mortality. Dr. Frances Rothert, under the auspices of the Children's Bureau, analyzed the maternal mortality figures from fifteen states and determined that the absence of prenatal care was a common factor in each case of maternal death. Of rural black women, 83 percent had no prenatal care and 13 percent had what was classified as inadequate care.[23] This report published in 1934, based on mortality figures of 1927–1928, strongly reinforced the urgent need for the provision of consistent maternity care starting with the onset of pregnancy. Sadly, a decade later roughly 70 percent of all maternal deaths in Alabama occurred in women who had received no prenatal care, and 82 percent of all fatalities were of women who had attended fewer than two clinic visits, designated as inadequate care. The fact that poor rural women were dying at higher rates indicated that state departments of health needed to establish a service that could effectively reach isolated, largely ignored communities. Physician proponents of maternal health in Alabama urged counties to establish clinics as one of the "surest ways" of improving maternity care and recommended that each and every county appoint a chairman of maternal and child health for a five-year term.[24] However, such oversight took a degree of dedication and expense that was inconsistent across each state and the region as a whole. In 1950, with one of the highest maternal mortality rates in the nation, Alabama reported twenty-seven counties still "refusing" to institute any form of prenatal service for its poorest citizens. Given the success of the state's Macon County nurse-midwife supervisory program such resistance is difficult to unravel. However, Dr. Thomas Boulware, associate professor of obstetrics at the University of Alabama in Birmingham and long-term representative in the state medical association, understood the essence of the opposition: indifference.[25]

CHAPTER 8

AFRICAN AMERICAN NURSE-MIDWIVES

The need to organize a supervisory force of nurse-midwives for southern states in particular was self-evident, and much of the stimulus came from MCA graduates holding positions in state departments of health. In 1942, two graduates, Kate Hyder and Etta Mae Forte, were hired as faculty and staff of a newly established school of nurse-midwifery, the Flint-Goodridge School at Dillard University in New Orleans. They developed a six-month program for nurses with two intakes per year, and two nurses in each class. However, with the graduation of the first class in June 1943, the school was closed ostensibly due to changes brought by the war effort, but rumors circulated that local obstetricians and the city health department opposed its existence.[1] The two graduates went on to work for the health departments of Louisiana and Mississippi.

As an advisor to the Alabama State Department of Health, Margaret Murphy, a 1933 MCA graduate, was instrumental in the establishment of a school of nurse-midwifery in Tuskegee. By 1941, four African American public health nurses from Alabama had graduated from the MCA School of Midwifery in New York and had begun to establish clinics and a home birth service in Macon County, Alabama, in preparation for the first class of student nurse-midwives. Under the auspices of the Julius Rosenwald Fund, the federal Children's Bureau, and the MCA, Tuskegee's program in nurse-midwifery was the first serious attempt to supply adequate professional maternity care to the poor, beyond the supervision and licensing of lay midwives. The school's principle objectives were to educate graduate African American nurses in midwifery, to reduce maternal and infant mortality, to study the specific problems of providing care in rural areas where medical services were not available, and to improve the service provided by the John A. Andrew Memorial Hospital at Tuskegee. Moreover, the school was seen as a "pioneer venture in negro education."[2]

The Tuskegee School of Nurse-Midwifery opened in September 1941 under the leadership of MCA-trained nurse-midwives, with Margaret Thomas

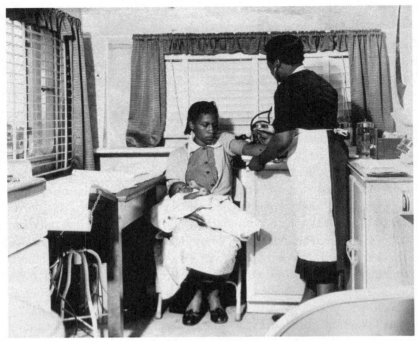

Nurse-midwife Eugenia Broughton with a patient at the Reformed Episcopal Church clinic, Berkeley County. American College of Nurse-Midwives. American College of Nurse-Midwives Records. 1946–1978. Located in: Modern Manuscripts Collection, History of Medicine Division, National Library of Medicine, Bethesda, MD; MS C 330.

as the curriculum designer and temporary director. Although fraught with problems of personnel retention, recruitment, and lack of real commitment from the Tuskegee Institute and hospital, the school graduated thirty-one African American nurse-midwives before closing in 1946. Its graduates provided a short-term supply of nurse-midwives, but many were seconded from their home states and had a commitment to return after the completion of the course. Moreover, the Bolton Act, enacted during the Second World War to subsidize tuition for nurse training, was available to applicants, but if acquired directly through the school, it merely obligated the nurse-midwife to use her specialized training for the duration of the war and six months thereafter; it did not stipulate that it be in Macon County.[3] Beatrice Trammel, one of the initial four Alabamian graduates from MCA, attempted to prolong the service of the Macon County nurse-midwife maternity service, but to no avail.[4]

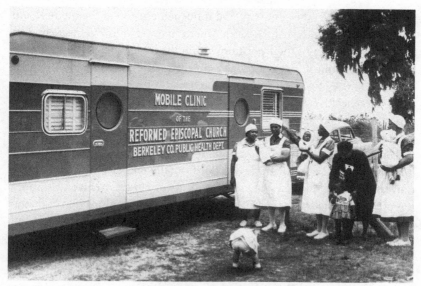

Midwives outside the mobile clinic of the Reformed Episcopal Church, Berkeley County. American College of Nurse-Midwives. American College of Nurse-Midwives Records. 1946–1978. Located in: Modern Manuscripts Collection, History of Medicine Division, National Library of Medicine, Bethesda, MD; MS C 330.

Despite its early demise, there was a significant reduction in the maternal mortality rate in Macon County. By its second year, the service delivered one-third of all mothers in the county with a mortality rate of zero.[5] By addressing issues specific to the community, the nurse-midwives working within a larger framework of state health-care provision were able to foster better relationships with the women and families they served. That women were happy with the care they received, and thus the effectiveness of counseling, is evidenced in the reduction in mortality that came as a direct result of early and consistent prenatal care.

But who were these African American nurse-midwives and how did they differ from lay midwives? Again the micro-macro lens is useful in highlighting the differences between the two groups of health-care providers. The lower social status of the lay midwives, although maligned by most in the wider medical community, afforded them some protection from racial and gender discrimination because their sphere of influence was at the grassroots, community level where they held a relatively high degree of authority; they functioned mainly at the micro level and so could avoid (by "flying under the radar," so to speak) the contempt and influence-erosion of the medical and state officials. In contrast, the African American nurse-midwives were middle class and, by virtue of their position within the larger society, came face to face with the almost insurmountable obstacles of discrimination imposed on them as they functioned within the broader framework of local, state, and federal health care. These macro-structural components influenced their experiences as professionals and as women, the care they were able to provide, and ultimately the longevity of the nurse-midwife service at Tuskegee.

Uncovering the precise fate of the Tuskegee-trained nurse-midwives is difficult; the Tuskegee Institute did not formally embrace it as part of the university and so neglected to preserve its history in the archives. However, it is possible to piece together information for about one-third (ten of thirty-one) of the graduates.[6] They were all dedicated and talented women, but some were predictably lacking in higher education because of the limited opportunities available to them.

Comparing Tuskegee's requirements for admission to those of the MCA reveals an immediate disparity between the educational opportunities for black and white nurses. The program in New York observed a rise in the preliminary educational level of its applicants, with 67 percent of all graduates having at least a bachelor's degree, but in contrast black nurses had very limited access to collegiate nursing education.[7] As late as the mid-1930s only one black college, Florida A&M, offered a bachelor's nursing program, and it was not until the mid- to late 1940s that the other schools followed suit.[8] The educational requirement for admission to Tuskegee was to be a graduate of an accredited school of nursing and preferably college eligible.[9] Of the more than one hundred training schools for black nurses only twenty-six were accredited by the National League of Nursing Education. Entry into these top-tier schools required high-school graduation, some of them stipulating a high class ranking.[10]

By cross-referencing the nursing education of the ten Tuskegee-trained nurse-midwives with lists of accredited schools it becomes apparent that the African American nurses selected for the program were superior candidates: well educated, intelligent, and some already highly accomplished.[11] For example, Helen Sullivan Miller, a graduate of University Hospital in Georgia, attended the Tuskegee School of Nurse-Midwifery after spending three years as a staff-nurse in the Georgia department of public health. She returned there as an area supervisor in maternal health in charge of midwife control. After a wartime stint in the Army Nurse Corps, she earned her bachelor of science in nursing with an emphasis on public health, before becoming the supervising nurse at the City of Philadelphia department of health. By 1957, Miller had her master's in nursing from Yale University and later became the chairman of the department of nursing at North Carolina Central University. She was the author of three books about nursing, particularly documenting the experience of black nurses, and was the recipient of several prestigious nursing awards.[12] Constance Manning Derrell, one of the last graduates of Tuskegee, worked in the maternity program in Macon County until 1949 and then became obstetric supervisor and director of personnel at the John A. Andrew Memorial Hospital. After earning a master's degree at Columbia University, she became the first certified nurse-midwife at the New York Cornell Medical Center Lying-in Hospital.[13] Influential nurse-midwives Mamie O. Hale of Arkansas and Maude Callen of South Carolina were graduates of the program, and similar achievements are not unusual for the Tuskegee nurse-midwives on whom documentation is available. Moreover, the focus on public health experience for admission clearly indicates the high caliber of Tuskegee's nurse-midwife candidates despite the dearth of collegiate nursing programs available to them. The optimal candidates were those that had at least one year of public health experience as well as one semester, or preferably two, at one of the just seventeen approved programs of postgraduate study in public health.[14]

While Tuskegee's program acknowledged the importance of public health education, such was not always true across the region, especially as it concerned African Americans. A census of public health nurses collected in 1926 revealed that of the 365 African American public health nurses in the United States, only 59 were employed in the South.[15] But the appalling state of general health of the African American population in the South did propel nursing leadership, black and white, to demand better state and federal funding for a greater number of better qualified public health nurses. To provide some perspective on the widespread need for public health funding, in 1932 a study by Yale University determined an appropriate per capita expenditure for public health to be $2.50. Furthermore, it advised $1.26 of that should be allocated specifically for child welfare and public health nursing. In Birmingham, Alabama, that year, the public health budget was forty-six cents, only nineteen cents of which was designated for public health nursing and child welfare.[16] One can only surmise how little of that was dedicated to the black community.

The time-honored theory that people of African descent had a predisposition for certain diseases such as syphilis or tuberculosis was giving way to the belief that ignorance and poor living and working conditions were more to blame than any biological weakness. Thus, it was concluded that in this field of nursing, one that emphasized education and self-help at the community, micro level, that the most effective work could be done if nurses were specifically trained and well prepared. Not surprisingly, the link between gaining advances for black families was tied to the impact on white families if officials failed to act. The medical director of the State Board of Health of Mississippi, Dr. Felix Underwood, employed his political prowess to promote more equality in public health funding. Using rational economical arguments focused on "enlightened self-interest," he gained support for his programs without challenging the status quo. He asserted that white health would be greatly improved if better care were taken of black people.[17] As Darlene Clark Hine observes in her study of black nursing, the urgency of protecting the health of white families in whose homes black women worked was a recurrent theme in black women's activism. In this case, that urgency opened a window of opportunity for black nurses to seize the initiative and make accessible health care available to their own communities.[18]

Once again, however, prejudice in the form of unequal education held back the pace of advancement. Despite the dire need for black public health nurses in the South, few black nurses held the necessary qualifications for specific study in the field because so few hospitals in the region met the requirements dictated by the National Organization of Public Health Nursing. This national body ensured that the general training curriculum included some emphasis on public health; also considered essential for success was the need to attract young African American nurses "with the best personal qualifications and background."[19] Members of this already elite group of public health nurses were selected to become certified nurse-midwives.

This group of nursing professionals was anchored in the "modern" healthcare system. As previously demonstrated, the nurse-midwives were the products of the best hospitals and schools of nursing, and the career paths of the ten graduates reveals the extent to which they were embedded in the increasingly centralized macro health-care system. Dr. John A. Kenney, in his address to the first graduating class of the Tuskegee School of Nurse-Midwifery, labeled the event auspicious "as it symbolized the transition from the old order in midwifery to the new."[20] He praised the unique coalition of the federal government, a philanthropic organization, a southern state, a southern county, and a "Negro" institution all working harmoniously for the development of midwives to serve the most needy of the "Negro" people.[21] Indeed, Dr. Kenney's rhetoric pronounced great achievement but in reality the nurse-midwives were forced to navigate a treacherous path. For the medico-political establishment, it was the nurse-midwives' social class and professionalism that elevated them above their race, allowing them a position, albeit tenuous, in a modern system. However, to optimally serve the neediest black communities, they had to subtly camouflage that separation and conserve a relationship based on race.

Tuskegee's program only began to prepare these pioneering women to negotiate the hazards associated with race and class. In conjunction with macro concerns about public health, as was typical with all nurse-midwifery schools, the program incorporated a focus on the micro elements of maternity care. The specially designed curriculum is a clear indication of particular emphasis placed on the specific, culturally unique, micro health needs of the impoverished black community in Macon County. Of the eleven hundred hours of instruction required to graduate, only two hundred hours were spent in the classroom, and just fifty of those were assigned for the anatomy and physiology of obstetrics. The majority of class time was devoted to the application of nurse-midwifery in the community, in pre- and post-natal care, parent education, and lay midwife instruction and supervision, with some emphasis on trends in current practices in maternal and infant care. Nurse-midwife candidates spent the bulk of the nine hundred hours not in deliveries, but on home visits.[22] Interestingly, in order to facilitate the provision of care to the homes of a widely dispersed community one of the prerequisites was that students knew how to drive. Furthermore, any student owning a car was requested to bring it with her, and if sponsored by a state department of health or private agency, she was usually eligible for a twenty-five-dollar-per-month stipend to cover the cost of its maintenance.[23]

As the curriculum suggests, despite their pioneering and modern approach to maternal health care, the nurse-midwives maintained some elements in common with lay midwives. Like the lay midwives who were culturally embedded in their communities, the nurse-midwives understood the importance of cultural awareness. The National Organization of Public Health Nursing promoted the replacement of white nurses by black nurses after a study revealed better results were achieved if "Negroes were met with the subtle understanding and sympathetic attention of nurses of their own race."[24] The public health community observed that this psychological advantage was essential to the success of any effort to improve the health of African Americans, and Dr. M. O. Bousfield, a vocal advocate of black health care, placed black public health nurses at the vanguard of this movement.[25] There was unanimous opinion that black nurses could more easily gain the confidence and trust of a community. One supervisor observed, "Negro

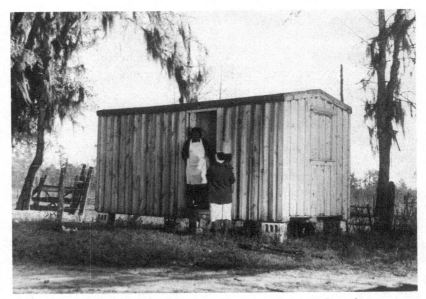

Nurse-midwife Eugenia Broughton (in apron) on clinic steps. American College of Nurse-Midwives. American College of Nurse-Midwives Records. 1946–1978. Located in: Modern Manuscripts Collection, History of Medicine Division, National Library of Medicine, Bethesda, MD; MS C 330.

people will not tell everything to a white nurse" and a black nurse is able to "gain the confidence of her people without reservation and understands how to overcome the peculiar superstitions of the more ignorant among them."[26] Like the lay midwives, the black nurse-midwives were more sensitive to the hesitancy of seeking medical attention.

Nevertheless, their education and professional background could not fully prepare the nurse-midwives for the environment in which they worked. Dr. Kenney in his commencement speech addressed the women as "frontiers-women with trained head, heart and hands." He told them that they would be thrown upon their own resources and that many times they would, while relying on their training and judgment, be "strained to their wits end."[27] He was right. For all their scientific training and expertise, neither Maude Callen working in Berkeley County, South Carolina, nor Connie Manning Durrell in Macon County, Alabama, were immediately equipped for the conditions they encountered. Most people in Berkeley County were tenant farmers with an annual income of less than $100. Their homes were often five miles from a paved road and virtually inaccessible when it rained.[28] In his highly regarded photo-essay W. Eugene Smith captures the incongruous image

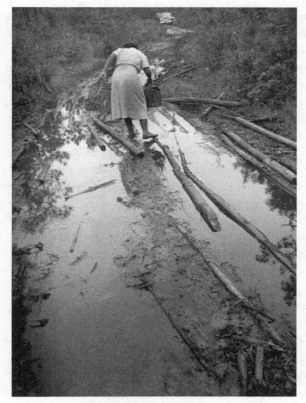

Nurse-midwife Maude Callen returning to her car after visiting a
patient's home, Berkeley County, South Carolina. Getty Images.
W. Eugene Smith, Contributor.

of Mrs. Callen, her bag grasped firmly in hand, wearing her neat uniform
and dress shoes, carefully picking her way back to her car along a flooded,
unpaved road strewn with logs and tree branches. This type of road was
typical in her 400-square-mile beat; at the end of some were found "people
who did not know the use of forks and spoons."[29] Similarly, Connie Manning
Durrell recalled her patients living in very cramped conditions; a home was
often little more than a single-roomed structure. "These homes," she reported,
"had no running water, no sewage system, and in many no outhouse!"[30] With
minimal equipment costing approximately $5, nurse-midwives performed
normal deliveries under aseptic conditions in homes such as these, the poorest most humble imaginable without sanitation or electricity. Like the lay
midwives they supervised, nurse-midwives were masters of improvisation.[31]

Certified nurse-midwives' awareness of cultural sensitivity was exhibited not only in their interaction with patients, but also in their relationship with licensed midwives. Lay midwives were treated with dignity and respect in their communities, and recognition of their influential role was crucial to the success of any supervisory and training program. An officer of the Division of Maternal and Child Health in South Carolina, when teaching comparisons between the modern midwife and her predecessor, always reminded the class of nurse-midwives to "never forget the granny because if she hadn't been willing and able to learn they [nurse-midwives] wouldn't be here."[32] Notwithstanding the apparent respect, there is little evidence to ascertain the universal opinion of nurse-midwives toward the permanent inclusion of lay midwifery as part of a modern maternity care model. In agreement with the medical establishment, Anita M. Jones, a nurse-midwife and assistant director of the Maternity Center Association, viewed the support of nonprofessional maternity care as merely a pragmatic solution to a temporary problem. In writing a teaching manual for lay midwives on behalf of the federal Children's Bureau she was explicit in the intended purpose of the manual, or rather what it was not: "It is not in anyway a textbook on midwifery, nor can the classes for midwives that are based on it be considered as 'courses in midwifery.' . . . Even when untrained midwives have been taught according to this manual they will not be adequately trained attendants at delivery."[33] Likewise Margaret Murphy, who was instrumental in establishing the Tuskegee School, asserted that it was "unattainable at any price" for all mothers in her state to have skilled care at childbirth, so her goal as midwife supervisor was to simply "improve the average midwife to a status of reasonable safety."[34] As professionals, it seems improbable that nurse-midwives would support the long-term continuance of a substandard service, particularly after they had effectively blended the essential elements of micro and macro care into their own practice. However, the component of race must be considered. In contrast to the opinion of Anita Jones and Margaret Murphy, who were white, the next generation of African American nurse-midwives actively celebrated their shared history with lay midwifery, so it is with caution that a similar sentiment is reflected back onto the Tuskegee-trained generation of nurse-midwives.[35] To the detriment of midwifery, though, a deep animosity between nurse-midwives and midwives of other backgrounds has persisted since. With that being said, the nurse-midwives of the mid-twentieth-century South were primarily assigned to oversee and train lay midwives, a task they performed wholeheartedly with respect and expertise, African American nurse-midwives being particularly effective in the isolated black communities.

CHAPTER 9

THE APPLICATION OF NURSE-MIDWIVES

A central tenet of the philosophy of the nurse-midwife was her role as an educator within a multilevel, interdisciplinary team. Nowhere was this more visible than in the midwifery summer institutes held each year in South Carolina for the training of lay midwives. Here, African American and white nurse-midwives formed an effective partnership with public health officials. The state's Division of Maternal and Child Health provided funding and organization expertise, with the nurse-midwives contributing their experience, clinical expertise, and cultural awareness. Midwifery supervisory programs such as these required a sincere dedication to improving maternal and infant mortality combined with a committed leadership at the state board of health; racial and economic barriers were enormous for even the most reform-minded leaders. The presence of influential and capable individuals at the helm was a vital component of a successful program: of note are Dr. Felix J. Underwood and Margaret D. Osborne in Mississippi and Dr. Hilla Sheriff and Laura Blackburn in South Carolina, who developed a particularly impressive service relying on two black nurse-midwives, Maude Callen and Eugenia Broughton.

However, not all states were equally dedicated to such schemes. As late as 1944, Arkansas still had no regulations in place to enforce adherence to the minimum standards of lay midwifery; a voluntary compliance with just five basic rules was relied upon with no instruction or supervision. The following year, under intensified efforts to reduce the disparity in black and white maternal mortality, the state board of health and the Arkansas State Medical Society drafted two recommendations. One unattainable option was to provide a minimum of five hundred additional hospital beds to accommodate the roughly ten thousand black births per year. The second more feasible suggestion was to enhance midwifery control, a process that was implemented in the summer of 1945 with the appointment of Mamie O. Hale as midwife consultant for the Maternal and Child Health Division of the Arkansas Health Department. A recent graduate of Tuskegee School

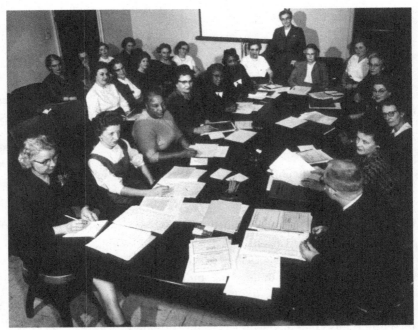

An interdisciplinary meeting at the Midwives Institute, South Carolina. American College of Nurse-Midwives. American College of Nurse-Midwives Records. 1946–1978. Located in: Modern Manuscripts Collection, History of Medicine Division, National Library of Medicine, Bethesda, MD; MS C 330.

of Nurse-Midwifery, Ms. Hale almost single-handedly instituted a program of education and supervision similar to the one put in motion twenty years earlier in Mississippi.[1]

Lay midwifery oversight in South Carolina was more in keeping with that in Mississippi. Beginning in the early 1940s in order to be licensed in South Carolina, in addition to their county-administered midwife club meetings, lay midwives had to attend a compulsory two-week residential course with a refresher every fourth year; new midwives were required to attend every summer for four consecutive years.[2] The Midwifery Institute was held at the Penn Center, a bastion of African American education since emancipation. Founded by Quaker activists on St. Helena Island in 1862, the school later adopted similar educational principles as Booker T. Washington's Tuskegee Institute with a curriculum of industrial and trade-based training. Struggling to survive as a school, the Penn Center reinvented itself as a community agency in 1948, and in addition to the midwifery institutes it provided space

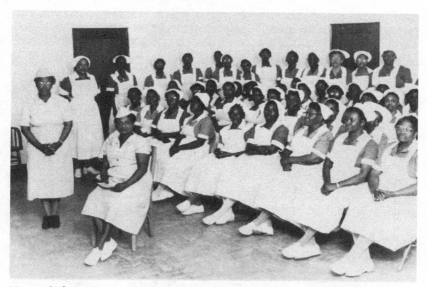

Nurse-midwife Eugenia Broughton with Berkeley County Midwives at the Penn Center, South Carolina. American College of Nurse-Midwives. American College of Nurse-Midwives Records. 1946–1978. Located in: Modern Manuscripts Collection, History of Medicine Division, National Library of Medicine, Bethesda, MD; MS C 330.

for such services as a community health clinic, a day-care center, and church retreats. It was an ideal location for the residential midwifery program with its classrooms, accommodation, and adequate kitchen facilities.[3]

Viewed in the context of the summer institutes, the gulf between the nurse-midwives and the lay midwives was enormous, and yet there was some blurring of the spheres of influence in the hierarchy of practice. Given the rarity of certified nurse-midwives, the most reliable and capable lay midwives, those who abided by state law and regularly attended the midwife meetings, were granted a leadership role at the institutes and at the community level.[4] Like the appointed midwife club leaders in Mississippi, group leaders like Mamie Stokes and Edith Baylor were handpicked by the nurse-midwives and were granted the authority to "preside over community meetings, dispense silver nitrate, inspect midwives' bags and ensure that any new members learned the revered Midwife Song."[5] Some helped nurse-midwives design activities to teach specific concepts. The selection of lay midwife leaders again demonstrates the nurse-midwives' tendency to focus on the individual, be she a lay midwife or expectant woman, to optimize the outcome. In the choice of midwife leaders, they homed in on individuals who

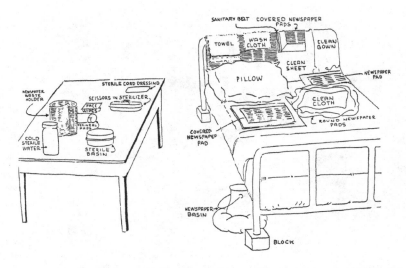

Diagram of room arrangement for home delivery in *Lessons for Midwives*. Dr. Elizabeth M. Bear Collection, Avery Research Center, College of Charleston, Charleston, South Carolina.

showed potential, reliability, and a genuine desire to advance midwifery. In the absence of a nurse-midwife, these top-tier lay midwives were trusted to reinforce modern techniques and standards of care to their peers.

Although the focus was on individual character, the real advantages of schooling were not overlooked, and so it can be reasonably assumed that the selection of leaders was directly related to age and education level; the younger midwives having attained a higher grade of education. Many attendees of the institute were taught to read and write during training as "few had more than a fourth-grade education."[6] Maude Callen and fellow nurse-midwife, MCA-trained Eugenia Broughton, were particularly influential in adding basic literacy to the summer programs in South Carolina. Midwife Josephine Matthews gratefully acknowledged that one unexpected aspect of being a lay midwife was that she earned a high school diploma at the age of seventy-four.[7] In a late 1950s sociological study of lay midwifery in North Carolina, Beatrice Mongeau researched the connection between literacy and success in practice. She concluded that having a literate body of lay midwives resulted in a more equal distribution of practice; an illiterate group tended toward a concentration of power in a single individual based on her personal attributes and skills.[8] In other words, literacy was associated with consistency and standardization. Clearly, a more equitable distribution of midwifery

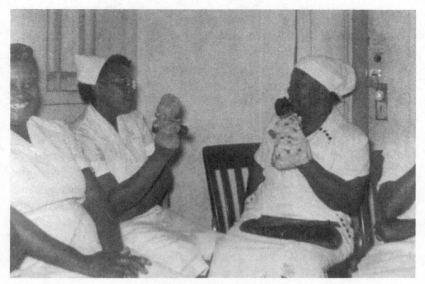

Lay midwives using puppets to practice dialogue in Clinton, Louisiana c. 1955. American College of Nurse-Midwives. American College of Nurse-Midwives Records. 1946–1978. Located in: Modern Manuscripts Collection, History of Medicine Division, National Library of Medicine, Bethesda, MD; MS C 330.

service better served the community, and that, in turn, validated Callen and Broughton's argument to include reading and writing in their program.

To overcome the discrepancy in educational levels the curriculum for lay midwives was thoughtfully presented not only at the South Carolina institutes, but in all states with a midwifery supervision program. Small classes of fifteen, preferably ten midwives were recommended for two reasons: to create an environment that encouraged questions and discussion, and to enable the instructor to properly demonstrate and observe each midwife's reproduction of a procedure. Demonstrations were particularly important to teach hygienic practices so classrooms had to be spacious enough to accommodate a realistic bedroom and kitchen. Attention to detail in the classroom ensured strict compliance in practice.[9]

Nurse-midwives developed a variety of culturally relevant techniques to enhance traditional methods. Skits and role-playing situations were devised to "ridicule" old superstitions and emphasize modern methods, and puppets were used to practice dialogues useful for educating women in the community.[10] Mamie O. Hale used a travel metaphor to describe the desired changes in practice. She coined the term *airplane midwives* to indicate that they were modern and had superseded the horse-drawn carriage. In fact, a midwife suspected by her peers of clinging to old methods was referred to as a "horse and buggy" midwife, an insult of the highest degree.[11]

Colloquial expressions and familiar terms replaced medical jargon. Simplified catchphrases such as "passage [birth canal], powers [contractions], passenger [baby]" were used to break down the process of birth into components.[12] Always having used the term "catching" babies, lay midwives were taught the mechanics of the second stage of labor by reinforcing the literal definition of the verb: "The baby is pushed out from above and the midwife should never do any pulling but should just support and 'catch' the baby as he is pushed out."[13] Always aware of the potential dangers of infection and hemorrhage they were taught to carefully observe the placenta and membranes on delivery. Medical terminology was replaced with obvious observations: "Note the color. Does it look like fresh meat or does it look dark and old and slightly decayed? Note the odor. Has it a fresh-meat odor or has it a spoiled offensive smell?"[14] The placenta is lobular and has the appearance of a pan of cooked biscuits and midwives were taught to ensure that "none of the biscuits were missing."[15] If any part was missing or abnormal, a physician had to be called as retention leads to excessive bleeding and infection. In fact, hemorrhage was a cause of maternal death that was particularly intractable.

Instructions and procedures were set to familiar tunes so that standards of modern care could be more easily taught and remembered, particularly by those lay midwives at a lower literacy level. An illustration of this is Eugenia Broughton's Birth Certificate Song that transmits the necessity of accurate birth registration. The Midwife Song featured regularly at midwife meetings, reinforces hygiene mandates. The lyrics, sung to the tune of "Mary Had a Little Lamb," describe proper dress and scrubbing procedure for delivery, and specific hand motions accompanied each verse.

Why does the midwife wear a wash dress?	(Hold dress)
Wear a wash dress, wear a wash dress?	
Why does the midwife wear a wash dress?	
TO PROTECT THE MOTHER AND BABY.	(Claps hands)
Why does the midwife wear a clean cap?	(Points to cap)
Wear a clean cap, wear a clean cap?	
Why does the midwife wear a clean cap?	
TO PROTECT THE MOTHER AND BABY.	(Claps hands)
Why does the midwife wear a clean mask?	(Put hands to face)

Wear a clean mask, wear a clean mask?
Why does the midwife wear a clean mask?
TO PROTECT THE MOTHER AND BABY.   (Claps hands)

Why does the midwife wear a clean gown?   (Holds out arms)
Wear a clean gown, wear a clean gown?
Why does the midwife wear a clean gown?
TO PROTECT THE MOTHER AND BABY.   (Claps hands)

And so on....
Why does the midwife clean her nails?   (Cleans nails)
Why does the midwife scrub her hands?   (Scrubs hands)
Why does the midwife soak her hands?   (Soaks hands)
Why does the midwife make paper pads?   (Measures pad)[16]

In keeping with the holistic approach to good maternal health, a hallmark of nurse-midwifery is their incorporation into an interdisciplinary team. Dietitians, mental health consultants, public health nurses, and doctors collaborated with nurse-midwives to review lesson plans and schedule activities to optimize the efficacy of the training. When interacting with black team members and lay midwives, white public health officers displayed a sense of pragmatism that frequently took precedence over the accustomed social mores of the Jim Crow South.

Relying heavily on African American nurse-midwives at the division of Maternal and Child Health in South Carolina, Dr. Hilla Sheriff, who was white, promoted an atmosphere of interracial cooperation. During a lecture by a visiting physician, Dr. Sheriff removed a screen that was segregating the audience. She argued that it overcomplicated the question-and-answer session that concluded the talk, explaining that the "doctor was a busy man who had little time for such nonsense." She highly valued the work of the nurse-midwives and despite being the first American woman to earn a master's degree in public health from Harvard University asserted, "I think I learned more about public health from public health nurses than I learned in any other place."[17] Dr. Sheriff's close professional relationship with Eugenia Broughton and Maude Callen, and the trust she placed in their judgment in developing the summer institutes, suggests that not only was she proud to include black professionals in her multidisciplinary team, but she also felt it important to afford them the recognition they deserved. Dr. William K. Fishbourne, the head of Berkeley County Health Department, agreed with

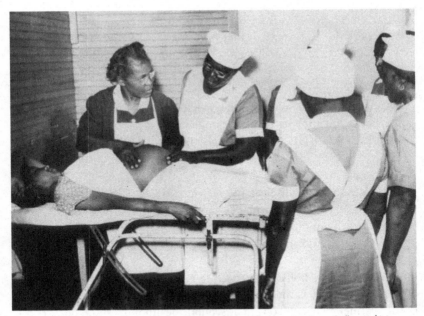

Nurse-midwife Maude Callen teaching a group of lay midwives. American College of Nurse-Midwives. American College of Nurse-Midwives Records. 1946–1978. Located in: Modern Manuscripts Collection, History of Medicine Division, National Library of Medicine, Bethesda, MD; MS C 330.

Dr. Sheriff's assessment. When asked if Maude Callen could be spared to do some teaching for the state department of health, the physician is quoted as saying, "If you have to take her, I only ask that you join me in prayer for the people left here."[18] With too few doctors to administer care, Dr. Fishbourne appreciatively relied on Mrs. Callen to relieve the burden of his enormous workload. Similarly, Tuskegee-trained nurse-midwife Mamie O. Hale was a well-known and respected figure among white public health nurses and obstetricians in Arkansas. In deference to her, Ms. Hale's white colleagues, when traveling with her throughout the state, boycotted restaurants that refused to serve African Americans.[19] Laura Blackburn, a widely respected white nurse-midwife who supervised and trained midwives for decades, constantly challenged social conventions in her work with African American colleagues. At this level of professional interaction, racial stereotyping could be superseded by reputation and character.

CHAPTER 10

PROBLEMS OF RACISM AND
CHALLENGES TO PROFESSIONALISM

Despite these apparently harmonious relationships built on a platform of respect and collaboration, African American nurse-midwives faced enormous
obstacles. The wider structural forces of legally sanctioned racial discrimination severely limited the long-term success of their services, and issues
associated with retention, recruitment, and funding proved to be overwhelming. Furthermore, the macro conditions of health-care provision largely
avoided by lay midwives were confronted head-on by black nurse-midwives
functioning within the larger medical community. Even within their own
profession they were excluded on the grounds of race. In the early 1940s,
the American Association of Nurse-Midwives (AANM), the precursor to
the modern American College of Nurse-Midwives (ACNM) held extensive
debates about whether to allow African American membership. Ultimately,
it was decided that whiteness was central to the AANM's conception of the
professional midwife, and black nurse-midwives were denied entry.[1]

Unequal educational opportunities for black nurses resulted in a restricted
pool of candidates for advanced training. White nurses had access to specialized postgraduate training; in the South black nurses rarely had such access
due to segregation laws. Even when appropriately qualified, black nurses
found it difficult to overcome the disadvantages of being paid lower wages
than white nurses. In Birmingham, Alabama, black public health nurses
were paid seventy-five dollars per month; white nurses, one hundred dollars each month.[2] They were openly discriminated against in the workplace
because of racial bias, and had to accept restrictions on housing and social
activities due to segregation. These problems were magnified for nurses at
the supervisory level.[3]

As an integral part of a professional interdisciplinary and interracial team,
the endemic discrimination they faced was intolerable to many. Even from
within the South recruitment was difficult, and acquiring students to fill two
classes per year was a constant challenge for Tuskegee's directors. During her

tenure as director in 1943, Margaret Thomas wrote to the director of public health in Arkansas advocating for the school. "The ground that has been gained in maternity work in the last twenty years will be lost," she implored, if nurses did not take advantage of the funds designated for nurse-midwife training. However, the availability of qualified nurses was equally limited in Arkansas, making it virtually impossible to establish any nurse-midwife service in the state at that time.[4]

The problem of recruitment and retention of high-caliber African American nurses in the South had long been identified by the National Organization of Public Health Nursing. A 1930 survey showed "a remarkable unanimity against accepting southern positions until conditions improve materially." The same publication put forth that northern nurses could not adapt to the "southern psychology," and southern nurses having completed advanced training in the North could not then revert back to the professional and social deprivations of the South.[5] Constance Manning Derrell returned to her native New York in 1949 after working for Macon County following her graduation from Tuskegee in 1946.[6]

She was one of the last nurse-midwives to graduate from Tuskegee School of Nurse-Midwifery. Despite meeting its objectives, Alabama withdrew its partial funding in 1943, the Children's Bureau subsidizing the difference.[7] Funds were eventually redirected entirely in 1946, thus ending the midwifery service as maternity care was restructured to provide greater access to hospitals. The Maternity Center Association determined the problem of retention as a significant factor in its demise. During the five years of operation, three directors resigned after a short tenure. As originally planned, six months into the program Margaret Thomas handed over her leadership role to fellow MCA graduate F. Carrington Owens. Although having a better academic pedigree than Thomas, because Owens was African American her salary was $800 lower. Even on appeal the salary was not increased, and she finally accepted a position in the North after a short stint in Tuskegee.[8] Three nurse-midwife instructors, all graduates of the MCA, resigned in 1942 citing that they were "all deeply interested in the program, but they could not afford to continue working under the unfair living and working conditions."[9] In an oral interview, 1944 graduate Nettie B. Jones reinforced this sentiment. After graduating, she worked as a nurse-midwife at the Macon County Health Department, and although she thoroughly enjoyed the work, her salary, which was lower than that of white nurses, did not meet her financial needs.[10]

The MCA assessment identified a lack of support from the Tuskegee Institute's John A. Andrew Memorial Hospital as a contributing factor in the school's brief existence, and reflects the ambivalence felt toward nurse-midwifery from within the black medical community. Already overburdened with patients, some black physicians like Dr. L. W. Long of Union, South Carolina, were relieved to see supervised county lay midwives. Long believed that in the absence of doctors they "did a good job . . . and there were very few cases . . . where the midwives couldn't handle the case."[11] For others, though, the promotion of midwifery even at a professional level perpetuated a "racial dualism" that was used to advantage by southern state boards of health.[12] Black physicians with the help of newly allocated federal funding pushed for a physician-centered, more mainstream health-care system. Although a welcomed intervention that modernized treatment and expanded hospital care, this approach toward maternity care solidified the concept of childbirth as a medical crisis, one that required the skills and scientific expertise of a doctor. A significant impetus to the shift in attitude was the wartime Emergency Maternal and Infant Care program (EMIC) that came in response to the medical care needs of servicemen and their families. During World War II, the gross inadequacy of the South's medical infrastructure, particularly in obstetric services, was exacerbated by the presence of a disproportionate number of military bases. In 1941, EMIC administrators, state departments of health, and the Children's Bureau negotiated an agreement to upgrade obstetric and pediatric services, thus facilitating a shift to hospital delivery. The absolute value of the EMIC to the African American population is debatable, but Dr. Paul Cornley believed it to be "one of the best programs ever developed" for black mothers and infants. He reasoned that since only families of the four lowest ranks were eligible for care, more black women must have been served because the number of low-ranking African Americans was disproportionately high.[13] The reach of the EMIC did not extend to the poorest of the poor who remained underserved by physicians and hospital facilities, but it underscored the value of hospitalized childbirth, and changes in expectation began to trickle down.

Beneath an overarching narrative of racism, for some African American women going to hospital became a marker of status; a midwife delivery was seen as an indication of exclusion, poverty, and backwardness; a hospital delivery, albeit in a segregated facility, a step toward inclusion within a larger, modern, and "scientific" society. Anthropologist Gertrude Jacinta Fraser argues that the pejorative racial stereotyping of midwifery effectively blocked any possibility of even a professional role within the South's medical hierarchy.[14]

From a micro-macro perspective, the work of an African American nurse-midwife reveals an approach to maternal health care that reflects current programs designed to promote better health-care access for black women. Skills of cultural competency are again considered to be essential in enhancing the quality of care, and the dissemination of knowledge via community leaders has proven to be effective in recent federally overseen projects.[15] However, within the context of the Jim Crow South, access into a strengthening system of federal health care was seen as a crucial step forward in the campaign for civil rights. Micro considerations of care were subsumed by an entry into a macro-level federal system that was perceived to employ fewer discriminatory practices and provide some degree of equality of care.

PART 3

CHANGING ATTITUDES AND BETTER ACCESS

Negroes of this area are becoming increasingly aware of ill health in members of the family before disease reaches an advanced stage, and come voluntarily to the health center for advice and treatment before hospitalization becomes necessary.

WALTER H. MADDUX, MD, ON THE SLOSSFIELD MEDICAL CENTER,
BIRMINGHAM, ALABAMA

The medical establishment was successful in its goal of transforming women's perception of childbirth from a physiological process to a pathological one requiring scientific intervention at birth. Ironically, though, as early as 1966, some doctors in the South were lamenting the state of maternity care. That year in an article in the *Virginia Medical Monthly*, an exasperated Dr. Gordon Jones complained that in "one month [he had] delivered twenty of these [poor, black] women he had never seen before, most of whom just dropped into the emergency room in labor, without having had any prenatal care."[1] The desired shift toward hospital delivery and macro-level care came at a price. The loss of familiar practitioners in the community who corralled expectant women into seeking medical care early, who ameliorated the derogatory climate of the macro medical world, and who advised and educated women prenatally, resulted in a negative change in behavior and attitude toward prenatal care. Nonetheless, once in labor African American women overlooked the racially demeaning attitudes and policies of medical facilities. With a growth in the number of hospitals during the World War II era, and hospital birth becoming symbolic of inclusion in American society, black women turned to hospitals.

The few African American doctors and activists who strove to bring some degree of equality to the separate health-care systems of the region also accepted the Western model of physician-led mainstream medicine. Influences from inside and outside the South eventually forced the creation of a medical infrastructure that brought modern, scientific care within reach, but the development of such a system was fraught with impediments grounded in racial discrimination and economic deprivation. However, the gradual inclusion of African American physicians into the professional medical body and the strength of federal mandates ultimately resulted in an expanding network of medical facilities and services for most. There can be no doubt of the enormous health benefits that accompanied this transition, or of the highest intentions of those instrumental in ensuring that the most vulnerable in society, both black and white, had access to modern health care. Nevertheless, in the final analysis racial, cultural, economic, and geographic factors inhibited some African Americans from seeking medical care even when facilities became available.

The prevailing theory that held sway during the mid-decades of the twentieth century was that medicine was a metaphor for progress. Huge strides were made in all aspects of medical research; with the expansion of knowledge and technology, hospitals became the center of practice, doctors became specialists instead of generalists, and personal attention was replaced by specific treatments. These macro components of health care reigned supreme over the individualized, trusted, and familiar components of micro-level care that functioned at the community level. However, it can be argued that these changes occurred generally, but not always in the direction of improvement.

Unraveling the complex web of obstacles that prevented African Americans in the South from accessing physician-led and hospital-based care necessitates going back to before the development of nurse-midwifery and well before the general acceptance of medicalized childbirth. Indeed, since emancipation, an assortment of issues created the intractable problems associated with African American health-care provision. It is a history of individual achievement as black doctors overcame the odds to complete medical training, and of collective endurance as black organizations established medical schools and hospitals. It is also a story of sacrifice as black institutions were forced to choose between perpetuating racial segregation by their very existence, or closing their doors in the anticipation of integration and equality. In the context of maternity care, it is a history that exposes the initial void that was filled by midwifery, and highlights the negative impacts of what was accepted as positive change in the childbirth experience of black women.

CHAPTER 11

OVERCOMING CHALLENGES

In light of high rates of mortality among African Americans in the South prior to the 1960s, it is not surprising that southern black health culture exhibited a persistent trait of fatalism. Folk remedies were widely employed when necessary, but denial of illness was reinforced by family or community pressure to fulfill obligations and responsibilities rather than play the "sick role."[1] Even when in dire need, medical treatment was sought reluctantly, and hospitals were considered to be places to go to die. If a medical facility was geographically accessible it was unlikely to treat African Americans, either because it was an all-white institution or because there was no availability of beds designated for black patients. In Mississippi, always the state with the worst ratio of hospital beds to its black population, there was less than one hospital bed available for every one thousand African Americans in 1938.[2] Moreover, the segregated black wards of hospitals were far beneath the minimum standards of the day in terms of cleanliness, care, and equipment. Added to this was the question of payment; dominated by a fee-for-service system, medical expenses were typically beyond the reach of the average black family. The experience of George Brown, a sharecropper in South Carolina, was commonplace. He never took any of his children to a doctor until one of them became desperately ill. The nearest doctor was eighteen miles away and across a bridgeless waterway. The fee for medical service was five dollars, an amount far above Mr. Brown's budget.[3] All in all, hospital care and medical expertise were simply not expectations of African Americans in the Jim Crow South, and they were largely unsought.

Black medical professionals and community leaders committed to solving the problems of black health care had many issues to address. Two of the most immediate concerns were the training and professional development of African American physicians, and the funding and support of hospitals to care for the black population. Success at dismantling these two mutually dependent problems was as important as it was difficult, since both required confronting institutionalized racism. The challenges cannot be overstated.

As Edward Beardsley observed, black physicians were "virtual prisoners of American racism and the segregationist structures it spawned."[4] At every turn their ability to practice medicine was curtailed by a wall of racial and class-based prejudice.

At the most rudimentary level of analysis, one problem was the limited number of medical schools open to African Americans. Some schools in the North and West used a quota system for accepting black students; the 1932 class at the University of Michigan was notable in that it included four black graduates, more than usual. Only two of fourteen black medical schools established after the Civil War survived into the 1920s: Howard University Medical School in Washington, DC, and Meharry Medical College in Nashville, Tennessee.[5] Between them they graduated more than one hundred physicians each year, but both institutions struggled under the discriminatory laws and practices of the South. Inadequate funding resulted in poorly equipped, antiquated facilities and the substandard education level of many entering students resulted in a high dropout rate and a low pass rate at the national board exams. The devastating effects of the Jim Crow educational system were evidenced in the fact that few students had the tools necessary to succeed in university-level and postgraduate study. One effect of this failure was to instill a sense of deficiency among those associated with the schools. As a graduate of Howard lamented, "We are daily made to feel that our diploma represents less and less in terms of solid, scientific medical training."[6] It was a dilemma for the administrators of black medical schools: would training greater numbers of second-rate physicians do more good for the health of African Americans than raising admission standards and reducing the potential pool of candidates? Since the schools operated on a tight budget, receiving fewer tuition payments could potentially force the institutions into closure, thus exacerbating the scarcity of black doctors.[7]

The numbers of black physicians did indeed decline in the 1930s and 1940s. With financial underpinning from philanthropic organizations such as the Rosenwald Fund and the Rockefeller Foundation, Meharry and Howard, no longer completely reliant on tuition payments, adopted a more selective admission procedure in 1940. The results were almost immediate, Meharry reducing its attrition rate from 68.55 percent of the class of 1940, to 7.69 percent of the class of 1945. But by the mid-1940s the number of black doctors graduating from medical school each year was insufficient to replace those lost to death or retirement. Approximately two thousand physicians practiced in the South, but they were generally concentrated in urban areas that supported a black population wealthy enough to sustain a private practice.[8]

Graduating from medical school was only the first obstacle for African American doctors. Their exclusion from most internships and residency programs for specialized professional training severely limited any career options. Most new graduates applied to the handful of black institutions: Harlem Hospital in New York, Provident in Chicago, or Homer G. Phillips in St. Louis, to name a few. Only those in the top echelons of a graduating class were offered the opportunity to be the first black intern at a prestigious white hospital.[9] Of their experience at Phillips Hospital in the early 1950s, Drs. Douglas L. Conner and Jim Montgomery recalled the realities of learning in a physical environment that was "not even as good as mediocre," while functioning under a staggering patient load with little if any supervision.[10] From the perspective of time, Dr. Conner, a general practitioner, came to believe that training under such circumstances enhanced his preparedness for practice; Dr. Montgomery concluded the reverse. Perhaps on a different career trajectory, Dr. Montgomery found himself to be ill prepared for the demands of internal medicine, his chosen field of practice. He identified the virtual absence of didactic teaching at Phillips as the reason why so few of his fellow residents in the 1950s were successful in American board examinations: "You see, you may well know how to diagnose and treat any problem, but on examination you've got to know about the chemistry of the problem, you've got to know about the physiology of the problem, you've got to know a whole lot of other things about the problem when you're going through multiple choice examinations." His experience at Phillips was brought into high relief later on when he contrasted it to the program at Beth Israel Hospital in Boston where daily teaching sessions were held with the professors. In Dr. Montgomery's estimation, the gulf between the two hospitals was enormous: at one, black residents worked on behalf of the city to treat black patients and prevent them from requiring admission to the white hospital; at the other, residents were taught to become physicians.[11]

With an internship or residency program completed, access to continuing education was equally difficult. Intractable rules of segregation severely compromised any attempt to attend conferences. Only because annual seminars were partially funded by the Commonwealth Fund did the Medical Association of the State of Alabama allow black doctors to attend in 1939. However, to conform to local sensibilities the lectures were repeated for a black audience, or failing that black physicians were required to leave the room for clinical demonstrations.[12] Twenty years later, while preparing to take his board examinations, Dr. Montgomery requested permission to attend grand rounds and teaching sessions at the University of Alabama Medical School in Birmingham. The doctor he asked was a faculty member, and despite the fact that the two men considered themselves friends, he was denied access.[13]

In addition, many black physicians were unable to gain membership to the American Medical Association. In order to join the AMA, a doctor had to be accepted by a local state or county medical society, but in the South, African Americans were excluded from the societies until the late 1950s. (Dr. Jim Montgomery was one of the first black members of the Jefferson County Medical Society in Birmingham, Alabama.) Compounding the problem yet further was the fact that membership in the AMA or local affiliate was often a criteria for a staff position in hospital.[14] Frustrated doctors argued, "It is impossible for a Negro surgeon to keep himself in good standing with the American College of Surgeons in the South, where local medical associations refuse to admit him to membership and accredited hospitals deny him affiliation."[15] In 1939, there were fewer than twenty-five black specialists practicing in the United States, and the challenges faced by black medical schools and the limited postgraduate opportunities for black doctors fostered a general perception that they were less well trained than their white counterparts. As Thomas J. Ward Jr. argues, it was an accurate assessment that drove even African American patients to prefer the attention of a white doctor.[16] Dr. Conner's experience may have aligned with Ward's statement to some degree; however, he attributed black hesitancy to seek out a black doctor to an entrenched belief of inferiority, a tendency he observed to be more prevalent in the middle classes.[17]

Beyond the impression of inadequacy, several other factors contributed to black doctors' guaranteed struggle for patients. The essential components for a thriving medical practice can be reduced to an equation: paying patients plus access to adequate hospital facilities equals a successful practice. Hesitancy to seek medical care and an inability to afford it on the part of the patient reduced the potential-patient pool, but hospital segregation laws that restricted a doctor's access to patients once admitted also impeded the growth of a private practice. In general, membership to county or state medical societies was required to gain hospital privileges, one function of the organizations being a screening mechanism to ensure legitimate practitioners. Although some variations occurred, usually black physicians were forced to transfer a patient requiring hospital treatment into the care of a white doctor on staff. Among the litany of foreseeable issues of granting privileges to black doctors was unwillingness on the part of hospitals to assume responsibility for fact-checking the qualifications of applicants. A significant fear for private hospital administrators was the predictable loss of white nursing and ancillary staff members who refused to take orders from a black physician. When placed in what was perceived as an intolerable situation, they sought employment in what was deemed to be a more appropriate working environment.[18] Small, rural, doctor-owned hospitals had the capacity to be more flexible, and yet faced similar issues when accommodating African American physicians. In Starkville, Mississippi, Dr. Conner was welcomed onto the staff at the forty-bed Felix Long Hospital in 1951. Owned by one of the town's four white physicians, the poorly equipped facility was of course segregated, but in Dr. Conner's estimation the care provided to African Americans was equivalent to that afforded to white patients.[19] A few white nurses showed disdain toward him by their slowness in following orders, but perhaps without an alternative option for employment in the small town, in general the white employees accepted his authority. To alleviate potential obstacles to delivery of care or hostility to Dr. Conner's ability, the hospital ensured that when on call, a white colleague supported him in case a white patient refused to be treated by him. It was an inevitable occurrence that Dr. Conner handled objectively and professionally; he calmly notified the other doctor on call, left quickly, and forgot about the incident.[20] He was guided by advice he had frequently been given by black people: "Go slow; take it easy; be careful."[21]

In some communities it was more than patient preference that restricted a physician's practice. Dr. Helen Barnes, beginning her career in Mississippi in 1960, ran afoul of a city law prohibiting black doctors from taking care of white patients. She became acquainted with the law when the Citizens' Council threatened action against her and her white patients should she persist in her violation of it.[22] A patient's gender could be problematic, too. In South Carolina in the mid-1950s, Dr. Ranzy Weston was surprised to be allowed to attend white patients in his segregated hospital, but there was one inviolable condition: his white patients had to be male.[23]

At the turn of the twentieth century as the medical profession became more scientific and standardized, structural racism intensified. Seeing little hope in making broad policy changes, the small but determined body of black physicians looked to themselves and their communities. African American physicians had established the National Medical Association (NMA) in opposition to the AMA in 1895. However, in 1923 amid growing concerns about the effects of the standardization programs of the AMA, the National Hospital Association (NHA) was created. Operating under the direction of the NMA, the NHA's objective was to support and maintain proper standards of education and efficiency in black hospitals. These two organizations are responsible for the survival of the black medical profession beyond the Jim

Crow era. The NMA and its associated journals and conferences provided an arena in which to fight the battle for integration of the profession and health services. By affording black doctors an environment in which they could gain clinical experience and training, the black hospitals and the NHA filled a crucial void.[24]

Black hospitals were either privately owned by physicians or established and administered by local fraternal organizations, but they could neither meet demand nor remain financially independent. In sixteen southern states, 9.7 million African Americans were served by only seventy-nine black hospitals, many of which were unaccredited, underequipped, and struggling to stay open under the financial constraints of serving an economically deprived community.[25] However, some stood out from the rank-and-file. The Afro-American Hospital of Yazoo City, Mississippi, was an impressive institution established in 1928 and managed by the Afro-American Sons and Daughters fraternal association. Its geographical reach is illustrative of the scarcity of services for African Americans; in a five-year period it admitted patients from thirty-three counties in Mississippi, and some traveled across state lines from Louisiana and Arkansas.[26] White philanthropic organizations such as the Rockefeller Foundation, the Julius Rosenwald Fund, and the Duke Endowment undoubtedly undergirded some black hospitals' fiscal stability, thus improving health services, but restrictions attached to the availability of funds created political animosity within the ranks of the black medical profession. The wide spectrum of opinion on how to best support black medicine is indicative of the complexity of the problem. Conservative physician leaders were adamant that an adherence to basic standards of organization and management should be a requirement for continued philanthropic support, even to the extent of adopting a white administration to meet those standards. The more conservative still expressed a need to establish white supervision of the medical services, too, as if in acceptance of white assumptions of black inferiority. Edward Beardsley concluded: "What was ironic was that they [the black physician leaders] were more conservative than some of the foundations they sought to influence." The Rosenwald Fund agreed with the idea of a white lay administration, but rejected the supervision of the medical staff arguing that black physicians would learn faster if allowed to manage their own services.[27]

Alternatively, African Americans requiring hospital treatment might find themselves in a segregated facility, perhaps one like Hillman Hospital in Birmingham, Alabama. Segregated institutions housed their black patients in overcrowded spaces served by inadequate amenities; at Hillman the black ward was in the building's basement where curtains separated the cramped bed spaces. Black patients were not unwelcome at such hospitals, rather their bodies presented a training opportunity for novice white surgeons. Dr. M. O. Blousfield of the Rosenwald Fund held the view that the provision of "material" for training was an institution's single motivation for admitting black patients at all.[28] Black doctors could not be offered internships to attend black patients in a segregated facility due to the presence of white patients, but it was a moot point as they did not have hospital privileges there anyway.

The crux of the dilemma of black health care lay in the hugely divisive issue of how to achieve integration: should energy be focused on improving black-only facilities, or should efforts be directed toward a greater inclusion of black patients in segregated hospitals? The promoters of black hospitals viewed the entirely segregated institutions as the only sensible strategy to gain a foothold in organized medicine and eventually achieve professional acceptance, and then integration. Many southern physicians agreed and preferred to bide their time and wait until the environment became more amenable to change; after all, they asserted, complete segregation was not ideal, but it was better than total exclusion. But by creating and accepting separate institutions, their critics accused them of condoning what was later referred to as "deluxe Jim Crow," simply a more palatable form of segregation.[29] At least by being present in a previously all-white facility, African Americans were in a stronger position from which to strike for full integration. As one doctor said, "It will be easier for us to come from the basement to the other floors than it will be for us to come from across town."[30]

The involvement of the federal government gave momentum to the proponents of segregating black patients in white facilities and undermined the fragile status of hospitals managed by African Americans and staffed by African American physicians. Change came in the form of the 1946 Hill-Burton Act that underwrote the construction of almost 500,000 hospital beds across the nation, and designated as a region of greatest need, the South received a disproportionate share of federal aid. It dictated that facilities built using Hill-Burton funds must not discriminate on race, but in those states where separate hospital facilities already existed for separate population groups, the nondiscrimination mandate could be ignored providing they "supplied blacks with enough facilities and services of like quality to meet assessed needs."[31] In reality, although facilities for black patients were better than they ever had been, they remained separate and usually unequal.

Hill-Burton's impact on the South was to spread the macro dimensions of health care in the form of hospital-based care, albeit in segregated facilities.

The George H. Lanier Memorial Hospital in Langdale, Alabama, opened in 1950, was the first hospital built under the new legislation.[32] Intent on upholding rigid segregation, a common practice of hospital administrators was to relocate white beds to the new facility and convert the old hospital to serve the African American community. In doing so, the hospital's governing body achieved two goals: more beds were made available for black patients as per the federal mandates, and the level of segregation was improved as black patients were no longer housed in a wing or basement of a whites-only hospital.[33] Where hospitals accommodated black and white patients under the same roof, a growing number of white patients saw no problem with the arrangement. Attention to modern designs and function created an environment whereby the two groups were kept in total isolation. On her release from a Hill-Burton facility in Raleigh, North Carolina, one very satisfied patient commended the hospital on her treatment received and accommodation. She went on to compliment the facility further by reporting that she "did not see a Negro patient."[34] Such a situation was the goal of Mississippi's sovereignty commission, whose role it was to enforce and maintain the edifice of racial segregation. In the view of one commission investigator it was bound to be "humiliating and embarrassing" for a white patient to be "subjected to constant association in the corridors [of a hospital] with Negroes."[35]

Cities invested Hill-Burton funds in large teaching hospitals that fostered the growth of institution-based, capital- and technology-intensive medicine. Such facilities served the urban poor as well as acting as tertiary care centers for rural patients, but the typical Hill-Burton project was a small hospital with fewer than fifty beds, operating in a community of fewer than five thousand. Forty-five health centers were constructed in Alabama alone between 1947 and 1962.[36] Improving access to macro elements of care began to alter expectations and attitudes toward health care.

However, if southern African Americans benefited from Hill-Burton to some extent, the same could not be said for black physicians who continued to be denied professional privileges at most hospitals until full integration was achieved in the mid-1960s. Those granted privileges earlier, like Dr. Conner in Starkville, Mississippi, tended to practice in areas where they posed little economic threat to their white colleagues.[37] When integration came, though, it swept in quickly and assuredly. Hospitals were motivated by federal funding and welcomed a future without the financial burden involved in upholding segregation; white physicians had no stake in maintaining segregation and many already had a professional relationship with their black colleagues. Black doctors were granted equal access to facilities, to specialists, to academia. In 1964 Dr. James Montgomery was awarded staff privileges at University Hospital in Birmingham, Alabama, and became the first African American on the faculty at the medical school.[38]

Unable to compete with financially sound, integrated institutions, black hospitals met their demise; once given the choice black people preferred to go to their local white hospital. Those that did survive the initial period of integration had failed by the mid-1970s or were absorbed into a larger hospital system.[39] The laissez-faire approach to regulation that had enabled fiscally poor institutions to survive came to an end, and state commissioners were no longer permitted to overlook infractions. The expenditure required to be in compliance with new standards of fire protection or bed spacing, or the need to install doors that swing both ways was crippling and hospitals closed.[40] Consequently, the careers of many older black physicians came to an end; having been denied advanced postgraduate training they failed to meet the educational standards set by the new hospitals. Like other black-administered businesses, schools, and institutions, integration caused black hospitals to fade away, as if suffocated by federal mandates that were implemented with the highest intention of support. Recently there has been a renewed interest in revisiting the benefits of such facilities to the African American community.

The experience of one black hospital suggests that present-day supporters are correct about their value. The Slossfield Community Center in Birmingham, Alabama, illustrates the potential of a facility of this type, one that blends micro and macro elements of health care, today considered so desirable. In 1937, a grassroots movement established Slossfield to improve community health, and its organizers took a broad view of health centered on "wellness." The hospital met general medical needs and addressed three specific areas of need: maternity care, venereal disease care, and TB treatment. Beyond this, the institution fulfilled the macro health-care needs by being "unique in the idea and practice of extending graduate medical training to Negro physicians."[41]

With its dense population, poor housing, minimal sanitation, and high rates of morbidity and mortality Slossfield was one of Birmingham's "blighted areas." To address maternal and infant health-care deficiencies, a maternity service was established in 1940 with funding from a slew of state, federal, and private sources. A ten-bed maternity hospital was opened for women determined to be high risk, and low-risk women were assigned to the home delivery service; patients were classified according to their parity, complications,

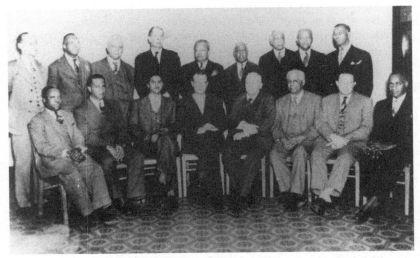

Dr. Tom Boulware with other physicians, circa 1940s. UAB Archives, University of Alabama at Birmingham.

home conditions, and accessibility to the hospital. The program was designed to definitively demonstrate that adequate maternity care does reduce maternal and infant mortality and morbidity. Furthermore, it intended to prove that with appropriate supervision and didactic teaching, African American doctors and nurses absolutely deserved full acceptance into the medical community.[42] Dr. Thomas Boulware, Slossfield's white senior obstetric consultant and vocal advocate for improved maternal health, reported the findings based on a three-year analysis (1940–1943): "We proved beyond any shadow of doubt that we could cut the stillbirth rate in half, the maternal death rate to zero, as far as true maternal deaths were concerned, and we stressed from start to finish conservatism."[43] The service made a remarkable impact: of the 1,168 deliveries, 80 percent of the expectant women had more than six prenatal clinic visits, the cesarean section rate was just 0.41 percent over the three-year period, and 69 percent of patients returned for their six-week postpartum checkup.[44]

The influence of the maternity service was felt beyond the physical boundary of Slossfield since a four-week residency program was offered to black physicians from across the state. Like the full-time residents, they received supervised clinical experience that was underpinned by regular lectures and discussion-based learning. It was the only institution to offer such essential training. Student nurse-midwives from Tuskegee were also required to complete a three-day observation at Slossfield, as were public health nurses. Reinforcing its regional importance, four-day postgraduate seminars were offered twice per year for doctors in Mississippi and Georgia, and Boulware taught obstetrics at Meharry and Tuskegee.[45] Furthermore, Boulware's political activity in the state and county medical associations ensured that Slossfield's successes were widely circulated among the medical establishment.

At the micro level, Slossfield's holistic approach to wellness connected good health to adequate housing, control of poverty, and effective support networks. To achieve these goals each patient was initially interviewed by a medical social worker; housing was assessed, as was employment and income; if the patient was unemployed, job training or education was made available, and childcare was arranged when necessary.[46] Furthermore, outreach health education programs were systematic and effective resulting in the community becoming "increasingly aware of ill health in members of the family before disease reaches an advanced stage," and individuals voluntarily sought advice and treatment before hospitalization was required.[47] This change in attitude was important in fostering a new expectation for care, a demand that grew in pace with increasing access as federal oversight of health care expanded.

Initially Slossfield was funded by local workers from the American Cast Iron Pipe Company who elected to have money withheld from their pay and by a grant established on the death of a local business owner. These funds were eventually supplemented by the Julius Rosenwald Fund and by a small grant from the Works Progress Administration.[48] As Jennifer Nelson argues, though, the increasing federal support for Slossfield beginning with the Children's Bureau support of the maternity service and later the Emergency Maternal and Infant Care Program came with a price.[49] Mandates forced a shift away from an expanded vision of well-being and community health toward a narrower, more mainstream emphasis on macro-level health care, and in particular, on hospital-based maternity care. In 1943, as it veered away from teaching, Slossfield became the only hospital in Birmingham to allow black doctors to admit their private patients. Community leaders and members of the governing board of Slossfield largely welcomed the increasing federal intervention because it ameliorated the racial discrimination from private and local public health services. Ultimately, though, funding was Slossfield's Achilles' heel, its financial support coming piecemeal from too many disparate sources. After being honored in 1940 as "the most outstanding Negro community center in the United States," Slossfield met its demise

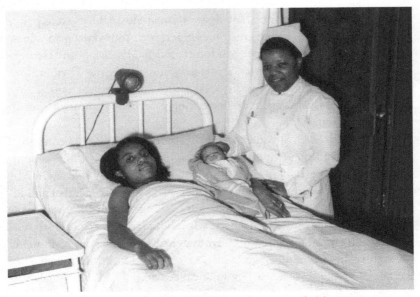

Slossfield Maternal Hospital, circa 1940s. UAB Archives, University of Alabama at Birmingham.

in 1948 when funding from the Children's Bureau was reduced and local agencies were unwilling to continue their support.[50]

As a local example of a broad, regional trend, Slossfield illustrates an important shift in African Americans' perception of maternity care. In its few years of operation it transformed from a black institution focusing on a sense of wellness, community, and self-help that is consistent with long-held African American concepts of health, to one that was increasingly under the protective umbrella of the federal government, promoting a more restricted vision of health. The desire for more inclusive, modern care trumped any concession for cultural recognition. Coinciding with the wartime EMIC, the physician-led maternity service facilitated the transition to a new "hospital consciousness."[51] By the time Slossfield closed its doors, the availability of maternity beds at Birmingham's county hospital presented black women with an alternative to home birth and when given the option they chose hospital childbirth, even if that meant seeing a white physician. In Alabama, by 1950 approximately 50 percent of African American women gave birth in a hospital (among whites, this figure was 97 percent).[52] Hospitals, however, were not a panacea.

CHAPTER 12

AFRICAN AMERICAN WOMEN TURN TO HOSPITAL BIRTH

As a trend then, for African American women in the South, maternity care made a rapid transition from home to hospital, from micro to macro focused. However, before the hospital infrastructure had expanded to accommodate black births, wholesale change occurred. Although rural black women continued to have midwife deliveries at home, they increasingly had some institutional health care. As midwifery licensing requirements tightened and mandated a prenatal examination by a physician, the reach of medicine extended to a significant portion of the population and maternity clinics were the entry point to macro health care. Dr. James Ferguson commended Mississippi midwives' success in this regard, and in a few counties of South Carolina, 90 percent of black expectant women were "given the privilege and benefit of a medical examination" by 1940. Access to the clinics initiated a more profound change; it instilled in women the importance of early and consistent prenatal care, and a higher value was placed on professional medical attention and medicine's authoritative knowledge.[1]

However, the medical profession did not always reciprocate black women's desire for medical care during pregnancy. Throughout the mid-decades of the twentieth century the unending clarion call from the medical association of Alabama's maternal health committee was the demand that every county organize prenatal clinics for all women regardless of race or class. In 1935 the committee admonished county health officers to "seek out every white pregnancy" so as to prevent these women from falling victim to black midwives. It was thought unconscionable that during the previous year, six thousand white women had been "forced to look at this blind empirical method of obstetric care."[2] The uneven distribution of African Americans across Alabama created so-called problem counties where a vast majority of residents were black. At most only two or three white general practitioners could sustain a practice in such economically deprived counties, and certainly no black doctors could survive. Time and time again, the maternal

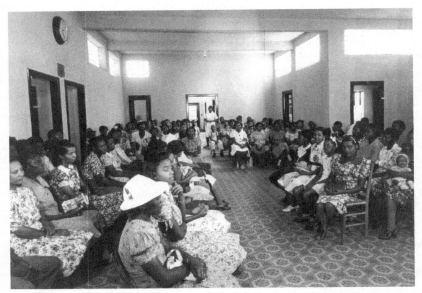

Slossfield Clinic, circa 1940s. UAB Archives, University of Alabama at Birmingham.

and infant welfare committee berated the medical community for their lack of foresight in addressing the needs of the poor. The suggestion of a partial payment system for white physicians or full subsidies to black physicians to attend poor black women in these counties was considered by many to be tantamount to socialized medicine and rejected entirely. In the meantime, professional maternity care was geographically inconsistent and the presence of active lay midwives continued to be acknowledged as a necessary evil.

A maternal mortality study spearheaded by Dr. Thomas Boulware illustrated the disparities and amplified his demand for action. Lowndes County, a "problem" county, where 90 percent of all live births were black, had the highest maternal mortality rate. Of those deliveries, just 3 percent were attended by one of the three white physicians in the county; they delivered 89 percent of white women. Admittedly, there was a single antenatal clinic, and as Boulware conceded, the doctors were willing to cooperate with the county and state health departments should a feasible suggestion be made. In contrast, Cullman County's live births were 99 percent white, and one of the twenty white physicians there delivered almost all of them. It had been the site of a successful six-year experimental maternity program established to emphasize early and consistent medical care throughout pregnancy. Boulware's study coincided with the termination of the program, with almost

94 percent of women receiving prenatal care, up from roughly 50 percent at the onset in 1938. The absence of a designated clinic in Cullman County supports the growing perception that prenatal clinic was a service for the poor and black. Significantly, the study exposed the fact that midwifery was not entirely culpable for the dire state of maternity care. In Jefferson County, where 97 percent of black women were delivered by physicians, where eight large hospitals, nine smaller institutions, and eight clinics served an increasingly urban population, one would expect the maternal mortality to be the lowest in the state. It was not: its rank of seventeenth of sixty-seven counties underlined the deficiencies in all aspects of obstetric care, and spoke to Boulware's point.[3]

Help came from an injection of federal funding for health care in the prewar years that reduced the financial burden on states and diminished the influence of discriminatory local policies. The Emergency Maternal and Infant Care program quickly followed and not only did clinics increase in number, but also the two–three-day-per-week mobile clinics were upgraded to permanent facilities. By 1950 the number of black women seen in Georgia and the Carolinas' maternity clinics was reportedly about fifteen times greater than the number of white; for better or worse, the clinics, like midwifery, became identified as a "colored" institution. It was a pattern seen across the South, and for many white women this negative connotation was an effective obstacle to care.[4] Unlike black women who were under instruction from their midwife to attend clinic, white women as patients of physicians felt no pressure to go.

Then as now, the importance of prenatal care cannot be overstated but not all clinics were equal in their efficacy. From the perspective of rural black women, it was likely to be her entrée to the modern and scientific, to macro health care; from the perspective of white public health workers, clinic may have presented a new type of interaction with those of a different race and class. Stereotypical assumptions created a macro-care experience that was less than satisfactory, and racism countered what was ostensibly an advance in health care. Paul Cornely, a black activist and physician, assessed health services in the South just after the Second World War and observed, "Negro patients were often treated with condescension, lack of sympathy, without respect and dignity, and without attention to many of the minor details for personal comfort and privacy."[5] The disdain for the patient was sometimes so great as to prevent the physical contact required in performing a basic examination. Some black physicians and public health nurses may have also struggled to overcome their own bias against the poor and hopeless patient.[6]

In the realm of macro health care, the relationship between practitioner and patient was less than optimal. The social distance between the two allowed for the intervention of prevailing negative assumptions of race, class, and gender, all intensified by an ignorance of culturally specific motifs and attitudes. The presence of lay midwives in clinics mitigated these issues to some extent, smoothing out the transition between micro and macro spheres of care, as did the presence of black nurse-midwives and public health nurses. However, the racism lessened the impact of health agencies as African Americans were less inclined to take initiative for their personal health. Moreover, it had the potential to damage relationships between black communities and local boards of health.[7] Nonetheless, black expectant mothers flocked into maternity clinics during the 1940s and 1950s eagerly accessing a more modern, scientific approach to pregnancy and childbirth. With few facilities per county and little or no public transportation, those without access to a car simply walked to procure the health care they chose.[8]

As the potential for physician management of pregnancy, albeit limited, became a reality for many women, and midwifery standards were raised under the guidance of local boards of health, the persistently higher rate of death for black women presented a conundrum. In assigning blame the focus continued to fall on the inadequacies of the midwife, but to deflect criticism away from themselves physicians shifted the responsibility onto the shoulders of the women. In her anthropological study of a rural African American community in Virginia, Gertrude Jacinta Fraser suggests that placing blame onto women who had received no prenatal care was a racially motivated way for physicians to excuse themselves in cases of medical neglect. A 1942 investigative commission in Virginia's state hospitals generally classified African American maternal deaths as "a preventable obstetric death because of the absence of prenatal care and the failure to seek medical help in a timely fashion. These failures were due to neglect or ignorance on the part of the patient and her family."[9] Other evidence confirms a false assumption on the part of physicians that black women were indifferent to their pregnancy and were "seldom willing to avail themselves of adequate care" even when it was available.[10]

Assigning racially motivated blame onto victims of childbirth did not obscure the disturbing reality of a physician delivery; the collection of more accurate details of maternal death exposed physician culpability. In Alabama, doctors attended three-fourths of the women who died in childbirth in 1933.[11] Their position in the "vanguard of transgressors" was due at best to a lack of understanding of obstetrics resulting in an inability to identify potentially deadly signs and symptoms, at worst to an unwillingness to adopt new techniques of asepsis or an absolute disregard for the reputation of their profession.[12] State medical associations attempted to educate those general practitioners doing most of the deliveries, but cooperation was difficult to enforce.

For hospitals in Alabama the mortality rate in 1939 and 1940 hovered around one death per one hundred and fifty deliveries; fully one-third of all deliveries was by cesarean section, during which approximately one woman in every twenty-five died.[13] Cesarean sections were four times as fatal for African Americans.[14] These statistics are appalling in comparison to the 0.41 percent cesarean section rate at Slossfield. As promoted by Thomas Boulware, conservatism was key and that required a level of competency and confidence that came with specifically educated obstetricians.

As the numbers of hospital beds gradually expanded, problems arose in the physical standards of maternity care provision. Some rural physicians argued that the home, under the supervision of well-trained and capable lay midwives, was a safer, more sanitary environment for delivery. Given the appalling standards of cleanliness found in black wards and hospitals it was an astute point that retained its validity until full integration in the mid-1960s. A 1930 survey of black hospitals by an NHA representative found some hospitals "so filthy and inadequately equipped and managed that one would hesitate to take a drink of water in them, much less submit to even the most minor surgical procedure."[15] Dr. Douglas Conner lamented that the facilities at Homer G. Phillips in St. Louis were "mediocre at best" during his internship in 1950. The confined physical space afforded black patients in segregated hospitals was hardly better, and cramped conditions limited differentiation according to illness. As Dr. Andrew Best recalled of his experience with a North Carolina hospital, "Whether you had pneumonia or a newborn baby, you were on the so-called colored floor."[16] However, consideration was often given to gender, male and female sections being simply separated physically or partitioned by a curtain.[17]

Childbirth under these conditions was uniquely problematic. Without a designated labor ward for African American maternity patients, the women were accommodated on a general floor where they labored alone, perhaps adjacent to a woman with gallstones, a diabetic with a gangrenous foot, or a patient recovering from surgery. When delivery was imminent, she was whisked up to the delivery room with time being of the essence. Inevitably many women delivered en route, in a corridor or elevator without medical attention, privacy, or dignity.[18]

Even when maternity beds were specifically designated for black women, conditions were little better. Complaints about a "Negro maternity ward" were published in the *Chicago Defender*. At the John Gaston Hospital in Memphis "a criminal lack of sanitation and wholly inadequate facilities" was reported in 1944. Trash-littered floors, standing water, and flies were commonplace, and the "newborns lying in box-like receptacles were wheeled about on unpainted, grimy wooden carts."[19] St. Martin de Porres Hospital in Mobile, Alabama, opened in 1941 to serve the African American community, but it had just four maternity beds until it was expanded to a thirty-five-bed capacity. Only then, in the 1950s, did it provide for the first time an opportunity for black physicians to treat their patients with "the aid of the diagnostic and therapeutic facilities of the modern hospital."[20]

What constituted a typical maternity care regime at the newly built facilities across the South is difficult to accurately assess. Certainly by the 1950s, the expectations associated with childbirth for most urban women, black and white, included effective pain relief and a medically managed labor and delivery that was conducted in a modern, clean hospital. For many African American women, access to scientific medicine and the macro health-care system represented an entrée into American society at large, and brought with it the hope for positive change. By distancing themselves from the negative imagery of midwifery and its associated poverty, black women put their maternal health in the hands of doctors and accepted the "appropriateness" of hospitalized childbirth as a better way to do things.[21] Although the number of black maternal deaths remained higher than that of white women, maternal mortality fell dramatically, the leading causes of death finally yielding.[22] Clinics facilitated the early detection and treatment of toxemia, more appropriate and timely intervention in labor reduced the incidence of hemorrhage, and aseptic technique became routine averting the risk of infection. Effective antibiotic therapy emerging in the postwar era was also critically instrumental in lowering mortality. Most maternal deaths were determined to be preventable.

Despite being safer and accepted as proper, scientific childbirth was reported to be highly unsatisfactory for all women, irrespective of race. Modern efficiency and sterility were equated to a regimentation and procedure that was reflected in nursing care during labor. Nurses were described as callous and brutal since they were the most visible agents of the strange and frightening routines imposed on women. In a robotic, mechanized way they separated a woman from her family, restricted all fluids, gave her an enema, shaved and swabbed her pudenda, and administered analgesic and amnesic drugs, rendering the women incapacitated and unaware of the birth. Laboring women were restrained at the arms and legs so as not to contaminate the sterile field, and left without an advocate for support.[23] The common assumption was that obstetric nurses and doctors were "mean."[24] Women who had experienced both styles of delivery, although appreciative of the availability of a hospital and obstetrician, lamented the loss of personal, caring, and understanding treatment. A woman delivered by Claudine Curry Smith commented, "The midwife was always right there and they was smoothing your hands and talking you. In hospital they laid you up on a table and nobody came in to see you until they think you probably ready for delivery. They put that cold stuff on you. They won't say nothing to ease your pain. The midwife stayed with you and held your hand and rub your forehead and they'd look and say 'well I can see the head,' you know, and then you figure out it was near about ready to be born, and it was comforting. They was interested and they was concerned."[25] The presence of a trusted practitioner was noticeably absent in hospital.

Apart from the lack of personal attention, access to macro-level care did not solve all the macro-level health problems for African American women. Even in a model of care that was impersonal and mechanized, black women did not receive the same level of care as did white women. According to obstetric nurse Faith Gibson, laboring black women remained on the general floor throughout the first stage of labor, and because they were not under constant observation by nurses, could not receive any pain relief. She also acknowledged the prevailing racist assumption that black women, as primitive and animal-like beings, had a reduced capacity to feel pain.[26] Despite his ardent support of Claudine Curry Smith and midwifery in general, Dr. Lamberth held a similar view: "I don't think the colored population really has much pain—the more sophisticated you get the more educated you get and the more you read, the more you worry, and the more pain you have. But they don't worry as much as they consider childbirth is a natural phenomenon."[27] And yet as Margaret Charles Smith observed, "These mothers, they still rather be in the hospital where they can whoop and holler, thinking the doctor is going to give them something to ease them pains, but the doctor won't be there."[28] When black mothers did place their trust in obstetricians to deliver their babies, evidence suggests that they were at a much higher risk of hysterectomy or surgical sterilization; one study revealed that 60 percent of black women in Sunflower County, Mississippi, had unwittingly had a postpartum hysterectomy.[29]

The increased availability of modern hospital facilities as a result of the Hill-Burton Act did not solve problems of access for all, as the affordability of hospital care lay beyond the financial reach of many. Edward Beardsley describes two very separate southern black populations to emerge after 1945; one increasingly urban, lying within the reach of public health agencies and private physicians; the other comprising of 35 to 40 percent of the whole who still lived almost entirely out of the existing health and medical systems, isolated in their impoverishment. The improving maternal and infant mortality rates that were largely seen in the first group gave reformers cause for optimism, but masked the true deprivation of the second group, a truth that was not revealed until the late 1960s.[30] The correlation between poverty and ill health was by then widely accepted, and yet institutionalized racism prevented the allocation of the desperately required funds when it came to black health care. Powerful physician resistance to anything but a fee-for-service system resulted in many, black and white, being excluded on economic grounds. Thomas Boulware was his profession's fiercest critic: "As long as the spectre of socialized medicine is raised as a roadblock to any constructive suggestion regarding the maternity problem of some of our counties, just that long will Alabama remain the 'here we rest' (on the bottom) state in maternal deaths."[31] In 1965 Medicaid brought promises of change, but in reality it was not widely implemented in most southern states until 1970.

In 1949, Michael M. Davis, the chairman of the Committee on Research in Medical Economics, argued for a national health insurance system that would allow poor people access to adequate care. Using figures published by the American Medical Association, he claimed that in 1947, 120,000,000 Americans earned below the minimum annual income of $5,000 required to cover the additional costs of medical care. More specifically, 75 percent of African Americans lived in states where the average per capita income was $1,000 or less, Mississippi registering an average per capita income of $555 in 1946.[32] These figures put into clear perspective the harsh reality of modern health-care access in the South.

However, despite the shortfalls in care and problems of affordability, African American women across the region became accustomed to delivering their children in hospital. In the postwar period, with the Emergency Maternal and Infant Care program acting as a catalyst, numerous factors contributed to the shift: changing attitudes, improved access, increased acquisition of knowledge and education, a rise in prosperity for some, a reduction in the number of lay midwives. Once more a focus on the micro and macro elements of health care is helpful in unraveling the subtle triggers of this shift. The situation in South Carolina highlights the important relationship between expectation and cultural change. In that state, beginning in 1940, the state board of health implemented and developed a sophisticated, efficient, and thorough program of lay midwife training, licensing, and supervision.[33] The successes were reflected in a dramatic improvement in infant and maternal mortality rates. And yet, although women were receiving a greatly improved standard of maternity care, within a model of care envied by other states, the shift into hospital was still decisive. According to government-issued statistics, in 1949, 60 percent of black women in South Carolina were delivered by a midwife, and significantly, given the level of state oversight, it can be assumed the midwife was a skilled licensed practitioner functioning in a multidisciplinary structure. However, by 1969, 90 percent of black women had a physician delivery in hospital. Women did not turn to hospital delivery simply because they assumed it was safer. In fact, in Alabama state records reveal a higher nonwhite infant mortality rate in 1964 than in 1955.[34] Clearly, the triggers for change were more complex.

CHAPTER 13

CHANGING CHILDBIRTH CUSTOMS

Beyond simply having better access to facilities and modern science, changes at the community level, the micro level, must hold more subtle explanations for women's shift into hospitals. From her fieldwork with elderly members of a rural African American community in the 1980s, anthropologist Gertrude J. Fraser observed that the actual and symbolic changes surrounding childbirth were largely understood as necessary to progress, and the loss of the midwife as an accepted exchange for inclusion in the health-care system at large. If progress and inclusion were associated with scientific knowledge and medicalization, then previously held perceptions of health, illness, and treatment had to be dismantled. Modern perceptions were strengthened by the constant accommodations and adjustments that occur within a culture, and lay midwives had played their part in molding childbirth culture to embrace the positive change that was initiated by supervision and the presence of local health-care infrastructure. The elderly women of Green River County interviewed by Fraser believed that medically managed births were more suitable for younger women as there had been a fundamental change in the physical bodies and sensibilities of women. It was assumed that bodies had altered in such a way that they no longer responded to traditional techniques and remedies, and the knowledge and belief of older customs were no longer transmissible from one generation of women to another.[1] Midwife Margaret Charles Smith came to a similar conclusion in her later years, observing that "the younger race having babies now don't be what the elder people, the older heads, used to be." She claimed that although some may learn from books, they do not have the capacity to learn how to be self-sufficient; in other words, they lacked "motherwit."[2] Customs involving a period of seclusion following childbirth eroded, reinforcing the fact that modern bodies were different as women seemingly recovered faster following delivery. It was accepted that scientific knowledge was more appropriate for these modern bodies.

Shifting childbirth customs in the younger generation was also influenced by the diminishing importance of social networks within the community. As the authority of the older generation waned, young women were less inclined to follow the advice of their mothers and grandmothers. Unlike the women of Green River County, some older women associated some new health issues with the failure to follow old-fashioned practices. For example, going out too soon after delivery, with or without the baby, was inadvisable. A former client of Claudine Curry Smith commented, "You stayed in the house for a month, not like the girls nowadays that has the baby, come home and they out . . . don't even stay in the house. I don't think it's a good idea because they're open and then should be careful lifting and all. But they go around doing the same thing they been doing before they had the babies which is not good."[3] Young women may have listened to advice given by older female relatives concerning diet, postpartum behavior, or infant feeding, but more often than not ignored it.[4]

By the late 1960s the implementation of Medicaid in the South ensured the certain demise of the midwives as the federal assistance program did not cover midwifery care. Many southern states structured their health-care plans in line with the political and economic philosophies they had maintained throughout; those being, a neglect of their obligations to the federal government, protection of a fee-for-service medical structure, and a disregard for African Americans and the poor.[5] In South Carolina, Medicaid coverage did not begin until birth, leaving pregnant women to arrange prenatal care and delivery at their own expense. Public clinics continued to offer care but became stigmatized as being only for the poor and black, and reached fewer women by the 1960s as emphasis and funding shifted away from community clinics to hospitals.[6] Women across America, not only in the South, were reluctant to go to the increasingly distant clinics because of the hours of waiting time, problems of child care, lack of transportation, and other poverty-related issues. Significantly, when interviewed they voiced the loss of the micro-level care, noticing that the doctors were disinterested in them, or the staff treated them disparagingly for being poor, unmarried, or having had "too many" children. The women admitted to being too self-conscious of their ignorance of pregnancy and labor to ask questions, and moreover, knew that any questions would be answered in an incomprehensible way. Anthropological studies show that women's dissatisfaction with prenatal care was translated into a relegation of its perceived value. The routine yet critical prenatal checks of blood pressure, urine, and weight were considered less important than the availability of a technological environment for delivery. Researchers repeatedly heard the sentiment: "As long as you deliver at a good hospital like ... you don't need all that prenatal care."[7]

In bringing desperately needed modern and scientific care to the South, the micro considerations of care were discarded in the name of progress, and African Americans adjusted their childbirth culture accordingly. The prenatal care that lay midwives had worked so diligently to facilitate became less emphasized partly because midwifery had lost its prestige, and there were fewer lay midwives in the community to direct women to clinic. In addition, women were reluctant to expose themselves to the negative experiences of institutional prenatal care, and its value diminished accordingly.

But more broadly, this progress was more than access to macro-level care, because by extension, it symbolized the inclusion of African Americans into American society at large, bringing an equality of access previously denied them. Yes, they gained access to modern facilities and physicians, and in light of the political and social context of the region and era, it is difficult to envision any other trajectory for maternity care. To their detriment, though, the lower rates of early and adequate prenatal care negatively impacted the health of their babies who were three times as likely to be of low birth weight, and five times as likely to die within one year of birth. The reality that many women face today must force a closer examination of models of care that existed in the past, ones that are more specifically designed with African American women in mind.

PART 4

MIDWIFERY IN TRANSITION

I'm worth millions of dollars for what I've done. I thought I was doing a big thing. I was proud of it. The lives I've saved going to deliver all these babies. . . . but they're losing a whole lot of babies now.

MARGARET CHARLES SMITH, 1996

African American lay midwives knew full well that their vacancy would be difficult to fill, and correctly anticipated where they would be missed. In fulfillment of the meaning of the word midwife as "with woman," the lay midwives were missed, not just in labor and at delivery, but as advocates for women throughout pregnancy, before, and afterward. They all endorsed what one elderly midwife argued: "They [midwives] sit down and talk to you how to do and what not to eat . . . they comes to see about ya 'fore you ever have the baby."[1] The midwives' manual stipulated at least three home visits prior to delivery and was explicit about education and prescribed topics of discussion at each stage of pregnancy. Even in labor at hospital, Margaret Charles Smith complained that doctors, at best, only entered the labor room in time to deliver the baby, and often it was the nurse who by chance just happened to be there. She argued, "You need somebody back there with you. Now a midwife, she's got to be right there, sitting right aside the bed or sitting over you, holding you, rocking you, rubbing you."[2] In the traditional communal sense of health and well-being, pregnancy, labor, and even motherhood were not experiences to be endured alone.

In the mid- to late 1970s, states across the South legislated against the certification of new lay midwives, but allowed those few still working to continue until retirement. In rural counties the practice petered out slowly as hospital delivery and access was not entirely widespread, and there was an increase in demand for home birth in the white community.[3] In Madison County, Alabama, fifty-seven lay midwife deliveries were recorded between 1978 and 1982, and the last being in 1985.[4] Although in full respect of the law and accepting changing childbirth expectations, it was difficult for lay midwives to completely withdraw from service. Convinced their skills were essential and their role extended beyond merely a presence at birth, lay midwives saw that their work was not yet done, and the needs of the community reflected this. Their role as educators and communicators, all enhanced by contact with the larger medical system, was left void when they were officially prevented from practicing. Their consistent presence, their role as liaisons, and their expertise on cultural mores were now removed from maternity care. The fact that women continued to seek the advice and wisdom of midwives, if not directly as a birth attendant, speaks to the importance of this larger, more nebulous role. Moreover, these facets of micro-level care that lay midwives performed so well were not reintroduced. Frustratingly, they continue to remain inadequate despite long-term studies that confirm their benefit. Macro-level systemic changes in the delivery of prenatal care have been ineffective in encouraging African American women to seek early and consistent care. In the United States only 63 percent of all black women begin prenatal care during the first trimester, and 10 percent either delay care until the third trimester of pregnancy or receive none at all; younger women and those with low educational attainment are less likely to receive adequate prenatal care.[5] However, success has been found in community-based strategies that focus on the individual. Improving family support at home and encouraging African American women to take ownership of their bodies and pregnancies have generated a more positive attitude toward pregnancy. These interactions are enhanced when they occur in a woman's community.[6] Just as lay midwives were instrumental in encouraging women to attend clinic in the past, some of their techniques should be rehabilitated to begin to address the racial disparities in access and outcome.

Certified nurse-midwives have filled the void to some extent, but because each state legislates midwifery independently they have struggled to challenge a powerful national medical profession for space in which to practice. Across the South, nurse-midwives are fighting to retain their scope of practice as state legislatures reinterpret laws concerning what is deemed to be appropriate physician oversight. In South Carolina, Lesley Rathbun, family nurse practitioner and CNM, has been at loggerheads with lawmakers in her effort to fulfill a new interpretation of what constitutes physician supervision at her birthing center, Charleston Birth Place, a site noted for its statistically proven safety for mothers and babies. In accordance with a long-standing law, the birthing center, located less than a mile from a hospital maternity unit, has medical personnel on call for twenty-four hours per day, seven days per week. In the rare event of emergency, the physician meets the nurse-midwife and patient on transfer to the hospital. In 2013 at the behest of the South Carolina Medical Association, the law was reinterpreted to mandate the physical presence of a physician at the birthing center to assess an emergency. Declaring the mandate unpractical and unrealistic, Rathbun explained: "In a true emergency which is actually very rare, we need the doctors to meet us at the hospital not to come here [to the birth center] first." A proviso allowing the birthing center to remain open expires in July 2018. Then, if not reinstated and the new interpretation is upheld, the birth center will be deemed noncompliant by the Department of Health and Environmental Control and be forced to close.[7] In fact, in 2014 almost 50 percent of the American College of Nurse-Midwives' fifty-five regional affiliate groups were active stakeholders in at least one legislative bill, and that is not to mention the action committees driving forward direct entry midwifery (midwives from a non-nursing background).[8]

Until recently much of the media attention directed at midwifery concerned the right for home birth. However, the high profile of a few very motivated and generally privileged women that demand home delivery should not obscure the needs of the many who currently have less than basic maternity care. Of late the popular media has focused on midwifery as a potential solution to the US maternal mortality rates. Of course, maternal and infant mortality is far lower now than it was in 1917 when the federal government was forced to react with the Sheppard-Towner Maternity and Infant Care Act, but as it was then, the United States figures are higher than those of other developed counties, and disturbingly so when the per capita cost of US health care is taken into account. Moreover, the racial disparities in maternal and infant mortality rates can no longer be ignored.

As the history of midwifery in America tells us, midwives are at their most effective in a much broader role during and after pregnancy, and the lay midwives self-appointed job description of "catchin' babies" is a wild understatement! Since the key to reducing maternal and infant mortality is found in enhancing prenatal care, it seems clear that midwifery with its particular skill set should have a place in an interdisciplinary maternity care system. Even if midwives do not currently have the political clout to compete with doctors in the delivery room, they certainly should have professional space during the prenatal months and afterward to do what they do best. However, legislative obstacles aside, midwives themselves have impeded their own advancement. As a group they have found it difficult to organize into a cohesive professional body, and it is proving detrimental to their progress.

Issues of professionalism, educational requirements, and standardization of practice have fractured midwifery into a multitude of subgroups, but there are some hopeful signs of cooperation with the ultimate goal of enhancing macro care with a modernized approach to addressing the micro factors.

CHAPTER 14

LAY MIDWIVES "RETIRE"

After decades of supervision and licensing, by the mid-1950s lay midwifery had adapted to the regulations dictated by the boards of health; midwives were generally younger, better educated, and better trained. Like Gladys Milton, who began her training in 1958, they were recruited into midwifery by the local department of health as the need arose.[1] They clearly understood their scope of practice and were well positioned on the fringe of the larger system to act as a buffer between the strange and the familiar as black women's expectations of childbirth shifted away from the traditional toward the modern.[2]

From the earliest days of supervision, the elimination of midwifery was to be partially achieved by the consistent elevation of the educational standards required for licensing. "Only intelligent midwives shall remain to practice," and so the selection of most suitable candidates, as prescribed by the medical establishment, began.[3] The strategy was to be "carried in the course of years to the point of practical abolition."[4] It proved to be an effective approach. In 1926 the department of health brought the midwives of a North Carolina county together for the first time. Of the 102 midwives who began attending training for licensing, all were African American, and only 56 percent were literate to the extent of being able to complete vital records accurately and legibly. Significantly, of the women under the age of fifty, 94 percent were literate; all over seventy were illiterate. The county eventually licensed only forty-eight women, generally the younger members, only one being over the age of seventy.[5] The early elimination of the most undesirable midwives was sometimes done with a degree of sensitivity, albeit from a presumption of racial superiority. In a 1931 advisory letter to the Florida State Board of Health, an officer acknowledged that their termination "should be made with due regard to their standing with their own people" and they should be duly honored for their services rendered, "faulty as it may have been in the past."[6]

Demanding basic standards of literacy for licensure reduced the number of practicing midwives, but the quality of maternity care improved and became more standardized. Another method was to weed out those midwives unwilling to adapt to the new regulations. Attention was directed to ensuring that rules and guidelines were consistently obeyed, and appropriate action was taken when they were violated. The penalties for failure to comply were usually enumerated in the midwife manual and depending on the infringement ranged from a fine of up to one hundred dollars, to imprisonment of not more than thirty days, to termination of practice.[7]

Despite occasionally creating a dilemma in the case of an emergency, as far as can be ascertained the midwives took the imposed limitation of practice seriously; like the women they served, the lay midwives accommodated to change. With the welfare of mother and child uttermost, they were fully aware of the potential dangers and as Onnie Lee Logan pointed out, "If I wasn't sure I would be in the biggest kind of hurry to get them [the woman] to a doctor."[8] Having seen two midwives stripped of their license for improper practice, and knowing one midwife who chose to stop working rather than function within a system of regulation and procedure, Margaret Charles Smith knew all too well of the power of the board of health to eliminate recalcitrant midwives. She told her friend at the clinic one day, "I'm through with them teas. They're going to have those babies with what the [midwifery] guide says, 'cause they [the public health nurses] told us not to try to help them."[9] Perhaps because she knew her midwifery skill could fill the void left by traditional remedies, or perhaps because economic pressures meant she was unwilling to jeopardize her paid job at the clinics, Mrs. Smith, like most midwives on whom there is documentation, followed the guidelines set by the public health departments.

The midwives' bag that came to exemplify the "modern" midwife was also the object via which their authority was literally and figuratively relinquished, in a similar way to a police officer turning in his badge. The regularly scrutinized contents of the bag were one indication of a midwife's compliance, and to be ordered to return the bag to the county health department was tantamount to being dismissed from service. "I had to bring my bag and my equipment in, not only me but all of them that was delivering," complained Margaret Charles Smith when notified of her compulsory termination.[10] By the same token, it was also an act of resignation. A midwife frustrated with the constraints of practice told her supervising nurse, "I think I'll bring my bag in and give it to you all because you all are not there when this labor is going on."[11] The same applied to the midwifery manual, always carried in the bag. It stated at the outset: "If for any reason you stop delivering babies, return it [the manual] to your county health department. Under no circumstances are you to give it to another person."[12] Knowledge formerly the preserve of midwives and transmitted by action and deed was appropriated, committed to paper, and was symbolically the possession of the state.

Anecdotal evidence from lay midwives suggests that although most accepted the legal restrictions on their scope of practice, they were less compliant with the rules governing retirement due to age. Having worked hard to maintain a license by following procedure, and attending the mandated midwife meetings and classes, some midwives were reluctant to retire when the time came. Before the late 1950s the spiritual component of the role was a powerful call to service, and an officially mandated retirement due to age was problematic; forced retirement represented a clash of the spiritual component of their traditional role with the secular nature of the modern role. When asked by the public health nurse if she was ready to retire, a midwife often replied with words to the effect: "My mind ain't told me. The Lord ain't viewed me to quit."[13] Retirement reinforced the control and oversight of the state, and the midwife faced severe sanctions should she decide to "unretire" herself. During the early years of supervision, elderly midwives, or those deemed unable to practice safely, were given the option of retirement while they were still in good standing with the authorities; some were pressured to do so. Later a more formalized retirement procedure was instituted. In Georgia, midwives were awarded a purple ribbon badge with the words "Retired Midwife" on the center in large gold letters. This was seen as preferable to a paper certificate of retirement because the similarity to a legal document was considered too easily "mistaken for a license to continue practicing."[14] However, in contrast, the state board of health in Florida issued a formal, authorized certificate stating that the midwife "has faithfully served the mothers and babies of the state of Florida, in the practice of midwifery and her service has been long and devoted; she has now voluntarily resigned from midwifery."[15]

In Georgia, a small pension proved to be a persuasive incentive for some midwives to step down; others needed more encouragement. To prompt action from midwife Aunt Jeanie, a special ceremony was held one Sunday at her church instead of at the midwife club meeting where many official retirements took place. Unaware of her imminent decision, she took her bag with her to church, as she always did. The service followed its usual format until the minister, a local doctor, commended Aunt Jeanie's work and leadership. After further testimony from several women Aunt Jeanie opened her midwife bag and held out her license to her supervising nurse. She announced, "The Lord has this day viewed me to quit and step down off the

Board. . . . And now if you got my badge handy, just pin it on me in the face of this congregation that knows I been passing faithful and never quit till the Lord knowed I can hardly get along, and He lifted all the burden He laid on me."[16] Some have called this type of ceremony coercive, and argue that the oversized retirement certificates and official purple badges patronized the midwives, but others argue that it provided the community a way in which to acknowledge a lifetime of service.[17] In Mississippi, elevation to the position of a Mary D. Osborne Retired Midwife formally honored retiring midwives, a title created out of respect for Mary Osborne, the long-term director of public health nursing and midwifery. As part of the Mississippi retirement ceremony midwives held small American flags. Taking into account their tireless work on behalf of the county and state health departments, the flags are perhaps illustrative of how the midwives perceived their role beyond the immediate community and an important recognition of their value to the nation, more specifically as American citizens.[18] These occasions provide another example of the boundary that existed between the micro and macro worlds, one that the lay midwives navigated so skillfully. The retirement ceremony afforded elderly midwives like Aunt Jeanie in Georgia and Josephine Franklin and Mollie Merrill of Forrest County, Mississippi, the opportunity to leave their vocation with their customary dignity intact, while simultaneously allowing them to satisfy their newer obligations to the state.

By the time lay midwifery was outlawed in the 1970s, most midwives knew better than to challenge the law, and yet they were not ready to willingly withdraw from service and continued to work for as long as possible. Although the demographic of their patient group was shifting to white, middle-class women, there were plenty of black women for whom lay midwifery was still the only option. Some were too afraid to go to hospital, some had been informed by the health department that they were ineligible for Medicaid, and some women simply turned up on the doorstep of a midwife's home in the throes of labor. According to Edward Beardsley's analysis of health care in the South, the haphazard implementation of Medicaid in the late 1960s brought little relief to the poorest 40 percent of African Americans.[19] Describing the plan as being "as much delusion as solution," he outlines the ways in which southern states developed innovative ways to limit access and circumvent the stipulations of the law. When enacted in South Carolina, Medicaid coverage did not begin until the moment of birth, leaving the expectant mother to cover the cost of prenatal and delivery care.[20]

The economic marketplace of childbirth, never a concern of lay midwives, was always an issue for physicians and became increasingly relevant with the expansion of federal reimbursement for services. However, an Institute of Medicine report identified obstetrician-gynecologists (OB/GYNs) as having one of the lowest Medicaid participation rates, a trend that persisted well into the 1980s. According to the report, in 1976, 63.2 percent of obstetricians served Medicaid patients compared to an average of 77.4 percent in other specialties. The reason for the lower participation was determined not to be the absolute Medicaid reimbursement for maternity care, but rather the differential between private reimbursement and Medicaid.[21] In other words, the financial rewards of attending insured patients greatly outweighed any need to supplement income by caring for women on Medicaid. It comes as no surprise then that in the mid-1970s obstetrics was one of the most lucrative fields of medicine and competition for insured patients was fierce.[22] This correlates with the experience of the surviving lay midwives who observed that once they began to deliver more insured white women physicians were consequently concerned about competition. In the Florida Panhandle by the late 1970s, 94 percent of Gladys Milton's caseload was white, and much of her clientele was well educated and had health insurance.[23] Onnie Lee Logan resorted to sending her white patients to black doctors for home delivery permits since white doctors would no longer issue them.[24] Mrs. Logan opined, "As long as I was doin' a lot a po' black girls they [white doctors] didn't care ... but when I started doin' a whole lot a white girls, nice outstandin' white girls, then that's when they started complainin'."[25] Gradually, all physicians stopped issuing permits (slips) for home delivery by a midwife.

Of the few lay midwives on whom we have record none understood clearly why they were being eliminated after decades of exemplary service. To be informed that they were no longer relevant was painful for the midwives whose emotions ran the gamut from betrayal, to sadness, to frustration. In 1980, seventy-four-year-old Mary Beth Chambers was given a *surprise* retirement party, but was never offered an explanation as to why she would not have her permit renewed. Under the circumstances, though, she admitted to being relieved. Uncertain about the new legislation and the withdrawal of midwifery support from doctors, Ms. Chambers worried, "I imagine you're gonna have to learn somethin' or other or do for yourself. 'Cause I understood that the clinic wouldn't be by you like it used to be."[26] Louvenia Taylor Benjamin was told that it was her age that was preventing the renewal of her permit; she was eighty, but was in good health and did not see her age as being detrimental to her practice. She was offended by the news: "I'll tell you. I never asked for a job in my life and I've never been fired off a job in my life. I said, as of today I quit."[27] Mrs. Benjamin was eventually invited to a meeting at the board of health, but since she was forced to conclude her practice she saw no reason to attend. In Virginia, Claudine Curry Smith delivered her last baby as a midwife in 1978, a year after the prohibition on new licenses. She retired from midwifery quietly in 1981, and as an indication of her good health and fitness she continued driving the school bus until 1987.[28]

Ensconced in their local communities in Alabama, Onnie Lee Logan was oblivious to the passage of the legislation, and Margaret Charles Smith's doctor with whom she had worked for decades continued his support of her because his patient load demanded it; he needed her help. Onnie Lee Logan only discovered that her license would not be renewed when, as per regulation, she called the board of health with notification of her three new patients that month. Mrs. Logan was furious to have been overlooked in such a way: "All a my good work that I've done. Didn't I deserve better than that? That long I've been workin' for the bo'd a health and didn't have any trouble." Her supervisor suggested that she write to the chairman of the board to request an extension of her permit for two more years; it was denied. She was a fit and healthy seventy-three-year-old, and fully capable of self-monitoring. In fact, she said, "If I start getting weak from my age they wouldn't have to pull me off. I'd just come off."[29] She was deprived of the opportunity to make that decision for herself.

If Onnie Lee Logan's experience suggests a gulf between the micro- and macro-level practitioners, Margaret Charles Smith's story is one of collaboration between the two worlds. Mrs. Smith and her local physician, Dr. Staggers, worked together for her final years of practice; he provided medical support, and after each delivery Mrs. Smith took the birth certificate into Dr. Staggers's office for him to sign and submit as if he had been the birth attendant.[30] In 1981, fearing repercussions from the Medical Association of the State of Alabama, Dr. Staggers called her to his office to confess that he could no longer keep her in practice. He commended her on her skill and compassion, and Mrs. Smith remembered, "Tears were in his eyes. He hated it so bad to see me go. I had to go ... that was the end of the midwives."[31]

In Florida, midwifery was also fighting for survival, but the more accommodating legal environment there had enabled Gladys Milton to open a birthing center adjacent to her home in 1976. After seventeen years of service across three states in the Panhandle, Mrs. Milton was delighted: "Instead of flying down the road in my old green station wagon to the tune of 'Move On Up a Little Higher,' I only had to walk through the den into the clinic."[32] She adapted as best she could to the tightening restrictions on practice and licensing for the birthing center, but she sensed an intensifying, more belligerent attitude at the health department after the passage of the 1984 Midwifery Practice Act. Her patients complained of poor treatment at the clinics when they attended for required blood work. One woman was asked by a young nurse, "Why in the world are you going to let that black woman deliver your baby? Why don't you just take your Blue Cross and Blue Shield and go to the hospital like every other normal person does?"[33]

At the age of sixty-four, Mrs. Milton received a letter from the Florida Health and Rehabilitative Service and was asked to retire. Taking the advice of a lawyer with previous experience of working with midwives who had been harassed by the state, she ignored the letter. Several weeks later she was informed of her options: she could retire or face "serious charges."[34] In a final act against her, the state sued for malpractice after she delivered a stillbirth. Ultimately, she was found faultless on all grounds, but during the ordeal she had an epiphany. She realized that the case brought against her by the Florida health department, the same department that had solicited her help as a midwife in 1958, and for whom she had worked so diligently, was not simply seeking to bar her from practice, its objective was to prohibit lay midwifery entirely. Despite being cleared of any wrongdoing, the health department disregarded the judge's ruling, and it was not until after a formal appeal that her license was finally reinstated.[35]

Midwives in Alabama were less fortunate as in 1976 the state legislature prohibited lay midwifery and criminalized the act of assisting at a home birth. This was a bitter pill to swallow for Onnie Lee Logan and Margaret Charles Smith. Having spent decades ostensibly following the guidelines that kept them in good standing with the boards of health, they now vehemently opposed their enforced termination. "All they wanted was the midwives off!" Mrs. Smith said, but the change in the legal status of midwives did not hold much relevance in the community where her personal authority was undiminished by the legislation. Women came to her in labor and one even delivered in her front yard. Mrs. Smith said she managed as best she could by accompanying them to a doctor, but typically the doctor advised the woman of the illegality of delivering at home, and promptly sent her home; on occasion the baby was born somewhere in between. One woman's mother said, "I started to Tuscaloosa. But my daughter was having pains so fast, I decided to turn around and come to you [Margaret Charles Smith]."[36] If Dr. Staggers was involved, rather than report Mrs. Smith for illegal practice, he simply instructed her to deliver the baby, ensure the woman was well, and then send her home. Onnie Lee Logan admitted to delivering one baby within three months of her license expiration. She was adamant: "I don't want no man stoppin' these hands from doin' what says the Lord. I don't need a permit to deliver no babies. If God tell me not to do it I won't do it." To circumvent the law Mrs. Logan declared that she would assist a father in the delivery of his baby. She proclaimed, "'Cause I don't go there to take charge like I was when I was licensed. I sit there and look at the father and tell him what to do and what not to do."[37]

Their duty to those in need was paramount and eclipsed any legal restriction. Gladys Milton attended a woman in labor who had been deemed ineligible for a midwife delivery. The woman came to Mrs. Milton in advanced labor and by the time she had called the doctor, who agreed that it was too late to arrange a transfer, the woman was ready to deliver. With no alternative Mrs. Milton safely delivered the twins. The Walton County Health Department reprimanded her for an infraction of the rules and told her, "If a woman that isn't certified by us is having a baby on your doorstep, you had better not open the door."[38] This was a preposterous statement because the obligation to help those in need was steadfast.

CHAPTER 15

MIDWIFERY BECOMES A WHITE WOMAN'S REALM

These few examples suggest that the midwives in Alabama communities retained a little more autonomy after their prohibition than did their Florida counterparts who were permitted to practice but within a heavily legislated environment. Certainly nurse-midwives, who had always been integrated into the macro health-care system, found the limitations of practice in some southern states almost insurmountable. The law regarding midwifery is complex and varied, but simplistically put, by the mid-1980s when the last African American lay midwives were retiring, states could be placed on a continuum ranging from one extreme, a prohibitory law against all midwifery practice, to the opposite extreme of no restriction whatsoever.[1] Nationwide, though, between 1975 and 1988 the number of in-hospital nurse-midwife attended births increased from 0.9 percent to 3.4 percent, but four of the five states exhibiting a decreasing trend were in the South, and the decline was concentrated among black mothers.[2] Nurse-midwifery became a small but expanding area of nursing that flourished more readily in states with a more accommodating legal environment, but nurse-midwives in the style of Maude Callen, Mamie O. Hale, and Eugenia Broughton were rarely represented in this new group of professionals.

The leadership of nurse-midwifery had been forced to make some contentious decisions since the profession's origin, the ramifications of which are seen in the modern face and function of nurse-midwifery. In many respects nurse-midwifery was presented with similar challenges to black lay midwifery. In keeping with the shift toward scientific childbirth, of enormous debate for nurse-midwives was their position in the macro-structured medical community and the degree of physician collaboration. The profession as a whole had to negotiate a fine line: how willing were they to sacrifice their position as autonomous practitioners on the frontier of nursing, in order to earn a respectable status and a position from which to grow the profession. Mary Breckinridge's Kentucky State Association of Midwives

(1929) evolved into the American Association of Nurse-Midwives in 1941, but the organization did little to promote cohesion or national recognition. Breckinridge was inflexible on professional ideology, and as a proponent of "slow growth" she advocated for a cautious approach that avoided conflict with physicians. Although recently challenged by some, Breckinridge's biographer, Melanie Goan, argues that race was also an area of contention in the early policy making of the AANM, Breckinridge being opposed to the inclusion of the forty-one black nurse-midwives, who represented 20 percent of the entire profession at that time.[3] Breckinridge's promotion of her isolated Appalachian patients as having a pure Anglo-Saxon bloodline and therefore worthy of assistance, and her promise to financial donors that her nurse-midwifery service would provide an "antidote to the forecasted weakening of American stock" among many examples, lend credence to Goan's assumption about Breckinridge's racial prejudices.[4] Despite some opposition by nurse-midwives trained and employed outside of Breckinridge's realm of influence, the AANM decided to proceed with a path less challenging to the medical establishment, and given the racial constraints of mid-twentieth-century America, whiteness was central to the profession's bid for a place in American health care.[5] The few African American nurse-midwives who had trained at MCA, Tuskegee, and Flint Goodrich were left without a voice as nurse-midwifery shifted toward the center of the macro medical system. Hattie Hemschemeyer from the Maternity Center Association was adamant that black nurse-midwives, many of whom were graduates of MCA, should be integral to whatever national organization was developed. Continuing to fracture along ideological lines, a new professional body was created in the mid-1950s, but it took almost a decade to formalize the group's philosophy and practice guidelines. With the death of Mary Breckinridge in 1965 came the amalgamation of the new American College of Nurse-Midwifery and AANM to become the American College of Nurse-Midwives in 1969.[6] Even though permitted membership, African American nurse-midwives, whose salaries were lower than their white counterparts, found the annual subscription fee for the ACNM almost beyond their reach. Maude Callen, for example, struggled to keep up with her dues on her monthly salary of $225.[7]

By the 1960s nurse-midwives were mainly working in hospitals with poor women in both urban and rural settings. As was the experience of lay midwives, the lower participation rate of obstetricians in Medicaid raised the need for nurse-midwives, and federal grants initiated by President Johnson's Great Society funded maternal and infant care programs for the poor that created an opening for nurse-midwifery. However, the hodge-podge of state- and physician-imposed regulations on midwifery practice and the varied educational standards and licensing status of practitioners created enormous challenges to the growth of the profession. In Mississippi, federal funds from the Maternal and Child Health Bureau were used to begin a nurse-midwifery certification course at the University of Mississippi in Jackson, but finding the required practical experience proved difficult for the nurse-midwifery students.[8] Joselyn Bacon, a 1978 graduate, recalled being prohibited from delivering babies at University Medical Center (UMC) in Jackson, the hospital affiliated with the University of Mississippi. To overcome this obstacle the program relied upon farming out the student midwives to other counties, even out of state. Bacon went as far as Baton Rouge. Even when permitted to manage deliveries, their practice was curtailed by local regulation. Bacon remembered being told, "Look, you can't do episiotomies because you're doing surgery, you can let them tear and sew them up, but you can't cut."[9] However, she did most of her clinical training in the Mississippi Delta town of Hollandale, where the university faculty supported a small county hospital and clinic.[10] Dr. J. Edward Hill began his medical practice in Hollandale in 1968 and seeing the dire need for a larger facility, he and his partner collaborated with the state to open a forty-two-bed hospital early in the 1970s. In 1975 he contracted with two nurse-midwives to support the high volume of medically indigent women and was enormously impressed with their ability as practitioners. In addition, the nurse-midwives designed and instituted a program for training local women to become nurse-midwife aides. Four aides, two of whom had dropped out of high school, were employed to support pre- and post-natal care in the homes of patients and were entirely supervised by the certified nurse-midwives. Dr. Hill recalled "not having much to do with the program" except he admired it as it relieved the heavy burden on the physicians. Occasionally the doctors in the isolated town of Hollandale had to refer patients for more specialist care, and there were obstetricians within a thirty-five-mile radius who offered support. Initially, Dr. Hill had a good relationship with his referral base but that changed when he began his association with nurse-midwives. Obstetricians neither referred patients to him nor accepted his complicated cases. He was forced to transfer patients one hundred miles to the University Medical Center in Jackson, though he admitted, "in a dire emergency they would see a patient but they made it very well clear that they weren't happy with it."[11] Dr. Hill's Maternal and Child Health Program made huge gains in maternity health and outcome, and routine visits during the first year of life produced an impressive reduction in infant mortality, and yet both the nurse-midwife program and the hospital were forced to close due to lack of funding. The school of nurse-midwifery in Jackson was also short lived. Only viable under the strong leadership of a single man, Dr. Theed, the chairman of Obstetrics and Gynecology, the school closed in the face of physician opposition almost immediately after he left the post.[12]

Similarly, nurse-midwives at the Medical University of South Carolina were constrained by local regulations forcing them to navigate a treacherous path between prioritizing women's health and following mandates issued by the chair of the department of obstetrics. The nurse-midwives were instructed to withhold prenatal care from private practice white women who had declared a commitment to home delivery with a lay midwife. At the same time, they were ordered to continue to see the mainly African American women who sought prenatal care in the public health clinics to clear them for midwife delivery at home. As the director of both the nurse-midwifery service and the nurse-midwifery education program, Helen Varney Burst found the hypocrisy of the situation intolerable, refused to agree to the mandate, and resigned.[13]

In trying to carve out a niche in mainstream health care, the American College of Nurse-Midwives issued a statement in 1973 that placed them in direct economic competition with obstetricians. The college considered hospital or an officially approved maternity home to be "the perfect site for childbirth because of the distinct advantages to the physical welfare of mother and infant."[14] This stance precipitated a heightened degree of restrictions from the medical establishment that denied hospital privileges to nurse-midwives like Joselyn Bacon in Mississippi, and supported state laws that curtailed nurse-midwifery practices. Likened to a selective county club, the administrators of one hospital told a nurse-midwife, "Let's face it, you are competition and we don't want you here."[15] In Alabama fierce opposition for advance practice nursing such as midwifery came couched in concern for quality of care. However, nurse leaders translated that sentiment into economic protectionism because physicians were amenable to nurse-midwives working in low-income communities but were adamant about limiting the birth practitioner choice available to middle-class women.[16] As proponents of nurse-midwifery argued, objection-based economic competition was without merit. In reality, physician collaboration with nurse-midwives proved to be advantageous as more patients were attracted to the practice.

The medical establishment was not alone in its dissent. The ACNM promotion of the advantages of hospital birth was immediately and vociferously challenged from within the profession itself. Amended several times before being finalized in 1980, the contentious statement is illustrative of the grow-ing disunity within midwifery. As the elderly lay midwives had encountered, the increasing disillusionment with medically managed birth came largely from white women, prompting a reactionary rise in interest in the practice of lay midwifery by white, middle-class women. These midwives generally came from a non-nursing background and were committed to facilitating home birth even if they were forced to practice extralegally. These more radical, nonprofessional midwives looked to the ACNM for political support and solidarity, but they were unsuccessful as they proved to be a polarizing force. After having worked tirelessly to separate themselves from the damag-ing image of lay midwifery, many nurse-midwives were unwilling to form an alliance with a nonprofessional group and risk losing the respect they had earned. Conversely, some nurse-midwives were afraid that they were already an elitist group and were rejecting their heritage as midwives.[17] The perpetual struggle that nurse-midwives have with self-definition and the concepts of independence and collaboration is both a strength and weakness. On one level it allows them to be adaptive, pragmatic, and resilient, when negotiating the structures of health care, and yet the lack of consensus on the fundamental principles of the profession is detrimental to its growth.

Irrespective of how nurse-midwives and midwives of other denomina-tions view themselves nationally, midwifery continues to be defined by state legislation that controls the licensing, standards, and scope of practice. To what degree an individual state views midwifery as part of its maternity care program is reflected in the rates of CNM-attended deliveries. In states where favorable legislation permits autonomous midwifery practice, mid-wife-attended births are higher; for example, in New Mexico one-quarter of all births are attended by midwives, and the rate is almost one-fifth in Oregon.[18] Moreover, analysis shows that women giving birth in states with a less restrictive environment had 13 percent lower odds of a cesarean sec-tion, 13 percent lower odds of preterm birth, and 11 percent lower odds of delivering a low birth weight baby compared to states with more restrictive policies.[19] Accordingly, states with policies more hostile to midwifery have fewer CNM deliveries with the lowest being Arkansas (0.56 percent), Mis-sissippi (2.2 percent), Louisiana (2.6 percent), and Alabama (1.67 percent).[20] Given the relationship between midwifery and better prenatal care, it comes as no surprise that these four states currently rank as the four worst in terms of infant mortality.[21]

CHAPTER 16

MIDWIFERY TODAY AND ITS POTENTIAL FOR TOMORROW

Almost a century after the federal government's initial foray into maternal and infant health and the licensing and predicted eradication of midwives began, midwifery in its modern form is poised and well equipped to improve maternity care should their numbers and the legislative environment allow. The vast majority of midwives today are certified nurse-midwives, and 94.4 percent of their deliveries are performed in hospitals, often to young, nonwhite mothers, and they attend more than 8 percent of all US births.[1] (It is worth noting that CNMs are now more relevant to black women as the few women currently seeking home delivery with a lay midwife are generally white and middle or upper class.) In a few African American communities, black and white CNMs provide a comprehensive care package, bringing together medical and social services at one location in a similar way to Alabama's Slossfield medical center in the 1940s. In many ways, the modern nurse-midwife interfaces with women as the lay midwife did, albeit from a position within the macro health-care structure. Like the traditional black lay midwives, an expanded role beyond the delivery room is prominent in their work. In fact, an African American nurse-midwife admitted that she rarely uses the words "I deliver babies" to describe her work, preferring instead to emphasize her wider role.[2] Primary health care is a priority that extends to counseling on health and nutrition, reproductive health, annual exams, and parenting advice. Family planning, or interconceptional care, was first introduced into CNMs' scope of practice in the late 1960s in a program transferred from a New York hospital to the Mississippi Delta. Today more than 50 percent of nurse-midwives identify reproductive health as one of their main responsibilities in their full-time positions, and a third consider primary care as a significant element of their practice.[3] The ACNM has expanded the practice of midwifery to include the primary care of women from puberty onward, a philosophy reflected in their motto: With women, for a lifetime.[4] A continuity of care and trust development, once a hallmark of the licensed lay midwife, has been embraced by certified nurse-midwives.

The relationship between maternal and infant mortality and prenatal care for all women is unequivocal; therefore, prenatal care for women at higher risk is paramount, and perhaps the statistical evidence says it best. The infant mortality rate for black babies is more than twice that for white, and in the Deep South the overall rate is generally higher than average with Mississippi topping the list. Significantly, the main cause of mortality in black infants is low birth weight from preterm birth as a result of maternal complications, in other words, problems that arise during pregnancy, many of which could be detected and managed if all women had access to effective care and understood the consequences of not seeking prenatal care.[5]

Getting women into the prenatal clinic is key, and was a problem managed effectively by lay midwives decades earlier by using education, by building relationships based upon trust, and by appreciating the woman in her broader context of societal situation and culture. Modern research into the triggers for accessing early and consistent prenatal care reveals some unexpected results and acknowledges the presence of tenacious cultural motifs in African American concepts of well-being and childbirth. Responses among African American women revealed a strongly identified relationship between spirituality and health, as well as the recognition of the value of kinship and support from older relatives. Folk health beliefs, such as eating habits during pregnancy and the danger of wrapping the cord around the baby's head by reaching overhead, were prevalent, and a distrust and general unease about interacting with physicians was still widespread.[6] At prenatal visits CNMs have been credited by women for taking more time with them, listening more, giving understandable explanations and information, and being more sensitive to questions based on culturally specific preconceptions, but beyond the prenatal months, midwives are again optimally placed to influence maternal and infant mortality.

It bears repeating that access to macro health structures is only part of the solution to providing satisfactory maternity care; socioeconomic factors add another level of complexity. Improving the socioeconomic circumstances of women is the most effective way to increase the rate of utilization of prenatal care. Teenage pregnancy, closely timed pregnancies, and an increased number of children are all markers of poverty, and the inopportune timing of pregnancies has been identified as a very high barrier to care adequacy. CNMs in their interconceptional role are well poised to intervene with contraceptive support. The presence of an influential maternal figure is effective in transmitting information to women reluctant to access well woman care, and again a CNM familiar with the family can focus her teaching and advice indirectly if need be.[7] By educating the entire community the certified nurse-midwife may facilitate the dissemination of information via older women to childbearing women. Nurse-midwife Heather Clarke believes that the preconceptual and interconceptual space is where real progress can be made. Community education, the initiation of dialogue, and control of risk factors such as obesity, diabetes, hypertension, and drug use *prior* to pregnancy will alleviate the cascade of problems associated with preterm labor and low birth weight infants. Thus, a proposal to develop a preconceptual model of care has the potential to break the cycle of chronic maternal ill health and poor maternal and infant outcome.[8]

Given the relationship between health and culture, and the incontestable evidence supporting the theory, the American College of Nurse-Midwives is acutely aware of its lack of diversity. Despite encompassing a holistic approach to maternity care, the cultural aspects of care cannot be optimally addressed given its current membership. According to Dr. Heather Clarke, chair of the ACNM's Midwives of Color Committee, although approximately 11 percent of registered nurses are black, less than 4 percent of CNMs self-identify as African American, and that proportion has remained unchanged since 1980. To combat the intimidation generated by the "sea of whiteness" that was the ACNM, an informal support group for African American members formed organically in 1972. For two decades black nurse-midwives met at the annual convention, usually in a member's hotel room, the time and location being distributed by word of mouth. Carol Ambrose recalled, "I got the whisper so I showed up."[9] Although informal, the "sisterhood" was cherished as an opportunity to debrief with fellow nurse-midwives who shared similar concerns and impediments to practice. Such stories helped to solidify this community. Shirley White-Walker, who eventually steered the group toward a more permanent basis, said of the early underground meetings: "I remember just being in awe of the people who had gone before me. I'm talking about Betty Carrington, Armentia Jarrett and various other ones who had to kick the doors in. I mean really kick them in."[10]

In 1992 the Midwives of Color Committee (MOCC) evolved out of an ad hoc intermediary panel, and significantly, that year the prestigious annual award for distinguished service was awarded to its first African American recipient, Armentia Jarrett. Furthermore, connecting her to a shared black womanhood in an acceptance interview Ms. Jarrett explained that her primary influence in becoming a midwife was her grandmother, Bettie Dorsey, the Mississippi midwife who delivered her.[11] The MOCC was charged with addressing the lack of diversity, and assigned to meet the specific needs of those of color, be they nurse-midwives, student nurse-midwives, or patients. The committee holds an annual closed meeting to encourage students and midwives of color to speak without reservation about their professional experiences, and each year they express concerns and complaints of institutional racism. In response, the committee established a mentoring program to help share the burden and relieve stress, and a scholarship fund to help mitigate the financial demands of nurse-midwifery education. The scholarship, now the Midwives of Color-Watson Scholarship, is large enough to assist minority students for the foreseeable future, and was first awarded in 1997.[12] Elevating the profile of its members within the college is an important function of the MOCC, and midwives of color are encouraged to present clinical research at each annual conference. Moreover, midwives of color have coordinated with the Federal Office of Minority Health to disseminate information about health disparities in order to raise awareness of the issue to the ACNM body.[13]

Many older African American nurse-midwives fear that merely maintaining a foothold in the profession is as challenging as growing their representation. A drive to encourage black women to consider entering nurse-midwifery was spearheaded by the MOCC, and to enhance recruitment established outreach programs to black nursing and professional organizations. Looking ahead, the ACNM has made the issue of diversity one of five competencies for its 2015–2020 strategic plan.[14]

The difficulty in attracting African Americans to nurse-midwifery is a reflection of deeper problems, some similar to those faced by black nurses in the 1930s and 1940s. Now as then, many nurses do not have the educational background required for master's level academics; only half of African American registered nurses have a bachelor's of science in nursing degree. In the 1980s when the master's degree requirement was first under discussion, the ACNM opposed the proposal on the grounds that it would be unduly restrictive since having a master's degree was proven to be unrelated to clinical competency. Ultimately, though, it was implemented as a vehicle to enhance professional status rather than to improve the quality of care.[15] Currently under debate is the further elevation of midwifery to a doctoral program that will certainly serve as a discouragement to many. Affordability has to be a concern with master's program tuition at around $35,000, and with an additional $12,000 for a bridge course to upgrade an associate's degree. The financial burden of joining the ranks of certified nurse-midwives is likely to be a keen disincentive even with the potential support of scholarship offered by the Midwives of Color Committee.[16]

So what options are available for black midwifery? Is it realistic to be singularly focused on increasing the representation of African Americans in nurse-midwifery given a thirty-year stasis? Not according to black midwives of all affiliations who are unanimous in their demand for new approaches to reverse the current trend affecting black women and infants. A groundswell of activism beginning in the 1970s and 1980s has been persistent in its attempt to preserve African and African American childbirth traditions. Black nurse-midwives supported these efforts and strengthened bonds between them and southern lay midwifery. While the ACNM wrestled for its identity and philosophy, Betty Carrington, a highly respected member who ran for college president in 1981, actively connected with the wider community of black midwives.[17] The tenacity of these movements is now coming to fruition as organizations like the International Center for Traditional Childbirth (ICTC) are receiving more mainstream attention. The ICTC, a nonprofit advocacy organization devoted to reducing infant mortality and promoting breastfeeding, recognizes centrality of the community in the efficacy of the traditional midwife and is taking steps to recreate that bridge between community and hospital, culture and science. In an ICTC pilot scheme the linear hierarchy of the macro health-care establishment is being dismantled so that lay childbirth educators from within the community can disseminate knowledge in a culturally specific way. In specifically designed programs, trained personnel cover a full spectrum of topics from emotional and physical changes in pregnancy, to options for pain management in labor. These models are neither new nor groundbreaking; lay midwives demonstrated that information presented by an individual who reflects the community and racial identity of the group and honors its culture and traditions is always more readily received.[18] Hollandale is a more modern example; Dr. Hill and his team of professionals and nonprofessionals illustrate how the micro and macro care can be integrated.[19]

Of great potential is the increasing utilization of a doula, a childbirth attendant, to fill the cultural void in macro-level care. ICTC oversees a highly esteemed doula training program designed to support prenatal, intra-partum, and postnatal women. Based in the midwifery-friendly environment of Oregon, the credential won approval by the Oregon Health Authority and doula care is now eligible for reimbursement by Medicaid there. Moreover, Dr.

Clarke with the Midwives of Color Committee has initiated a plan to partner with ICTC and is awaiting approval from the ACNM board.[20]

Elsewhere local childbirth advocacy groups are using doulas and trained lay educators to reintroduce midwifery to low-income black communities. As part of her practice, one licensed midwife and ICTC representative in Florida, Jamarah Amani, operates the Circle of Mamas program that "shares culturally centered health care information, including birth options and breastfeeding, in respectful, nonjudgmental language with pregnant teens." She and her team have seen successes in the longevity of breastfeeding, maternal bonding, and the improved self-esteem of the young women involved. Amani maintains that central to their objective is the reawakening of midwifery as an option in the youngest generation of mothers, a group of women who have had no prior exposure to their own history. Maria Milton, who sees few black patients in her birth center, hopes that through education and outreach, once young women regain a faith in their bodies' natural ability to endure childbirth, their fear will diminish in proportion to an increasing awareness of health, well-being, and self-worth.[21]

The principle distinction between midwives is their philosophy of practice and education, and generally speaking, black midwives committed to honoring and sustaining the legacy of midwifery in their community are licensed or direct entry midwives who may or may not have a nursing background. It is a midwifery model that most closely reflects the expanded responsibilities of traditional midwives and encompasses the spiritual and communal roles. The unwieldy array of state legislation, combined with multiple routes of entry and various midwifery credentialing boards, has generated a labyrinth of macro-level regulations, and when faced with navigating this system, a genuine desire to help the community and a deep, sincere spiritual inclination to midwifery may on occasion supersede the need to practice legally. This was the experience of Jamarah Amani, who began as an underground midwife, but quickly acknowledged that her ability to access the entire community was severely limited by her own illegality. Only through legal channels can midwives, community educators, and doulas reach out to high schools, seek reimbursement from Medicaid, and become incorporated into the larger framework of health-care workers. Positioning credentialed lay workers and properly licensed midwives at the grassroots level is the common theme of African American midwifery activism. Top-down adaptations in public health policy at the macro level have failed to filter down to those who are bearing the brunt of the maternity care crisis, but creating change from a bottom-up perspective holds more potential. Reaching young black women in their schools and churches, teaching their heritage of midwifery and community self-help, creating a local, culturally appropriate entry into the medical establishment has been proven to work. JayVon Muhammad, creator of SistaGirl Midwifery and CEO of Marin City Health and Wellness Center, admonishes her peers to unify, act on what they know to be effective, and document successes so as to enable replication in similar communities.[22]

In opposition to this micro-level focus, one could claim that it creates the same two-tier system that was dismantled with the desegregation of health care in the 1960s, one system reliant on trained, but nonprofessional black health workers, and one utilizing the full depth of expertise of highly educated, mainly white professionals. If progress is always linear and unidirectional, then surely it could be interpreted as a step backward. Dr. Clarke argues otherwise, but insists that a seamless transition between the micro and macro spheres is essential to success. Unlike the earlier scenario, cooperation, respect, and mutual appreciation must be central tenets of the philosophy of a maternity care model.[23] As history has revealed, even among midwives persistent conflict and lack of understanding has undermined their development and has the potential to jeopardize Dr. Clarke's hopes for a future built on shared goals and collaboration across a spectrum of maternity care providers. Very recently the United States Midwifery Education, Regulation and Association (US MERA) faced allegations of racial exclusion for failing to invite ICTC to join a steering committee comprised of seven midwifery organizations brought together to enhance cohesion. When initially challenged, US MERA admitted it had been an oversight, but moved slowly to rectify the mistake. In a statement US MERA announced that it was "evaluating" how best it might work with ICTC while staying true to its commitment to the global standards of the International Confederation of Midwives.[24] After submitting newly required documentation and the high-profile resignation of the only midwife of color on the committee, ICTC was invited to join the collaborative in February 2016. US MERA announced that it was "grateful for ICTC's passionate commitment to eliminating outcome disparities for mothers and babies."[25] Despite the inauspicious beginnings, the inclusion of ICTC must be seen as a positive step forward, and now, with full cooperation being aspired to within midwifery as a whole, the group can stand together to demand their collective integration into a multidisciplinary maternity service for all women, but particularly for those being disadvantaged by the current situation.

EPILOGUE

What better tribute to the African American lay midwives than to acknowledge that the hallmarks of their role were of legitimate value and not merely identifiers of obsolescence. Their lives and experience must be committed to the historical register, not as simply fragments of the past, but as potential tools for the future. As lay midwifery came to an end in the early 1980s, the few midwives that remained were eventually honored by their communities and beyond. For example, Margaret Charles Smith was presented with a lifetime achievement award by the ICTC, and was recognized nationally by the Congressional Black Caucus in Washington, DC; Gladys Milton was inducted into the Florida Women's Hall of Fame and her work lives on at her birthing center, the Milton Memorial Birthing Center, now owned and operated by her daughter, Maria Milton.[1] Yet the midwives were not validated by these accolades; they wished to be recognized for their commitment to their communities, their midwifery skills, their innate intelligence, and their ability to negotiate beyond their immediate realm of influence and become incorporated into a state maternity care system. As Onnie Lee Logan emphatically declared: "I'm gonna write a book even if I have to scratch it out." She did not intend her book to be an autobiography, but rather a testament to her "wisdom and knowledge." She exclaimed, "I want to show that I knew what I knew—I want somebody to realize what I am."[2]

Clearly, the growth of a macro-structured health-care system brought essential benefit to the desperately underserved population of the South; it is absurd to argue otherwise. However, as an exercise in historical analysis, a case can be made that the juggernaut of scientific hegemony forced into obsolescence a brand of care that held intrinsic value. It is inadvisable to approach the history of medicine with the intention of applying modern standards to the attitudes and assumptions of the past but, no matter how absurd it may be to argue against the benefits of modern maternity care, it seems equally foolish not to consider what was lost at the community, micro level, particularly at a time when a failing maternity care system is again creating enormous racial and socioeconomic disparities.

If granted the opportunity, midwifery may again come to the rescue of the most vulnerable women. Today the future of American midwifery lies in the hands of the roughly 11,500 certified nurse-midwives, the largest denomination of midwives. They continue to challenge obstetricians for a space in the American maternity care system, but their intention is not to supplant the physician, but to supplement.[3] The American College of Nurse-Midwives is faced with the task of growing the profession and achieving its goal of attending 20 percent of US births by 2020. In order to do so, it must also accept that it is just one piece in a mosaic of midwifery, and embrace the roles of certified doulas and lay educators, as well as midwives from a non-nursing background. As Helen Varney Burst argued decades ago, certified midwives must be inclusive toward other midwives, or else expose themselves to divide and conquer tactics from their opponents. Varney Burst promoted this approach during her tenure as president of the ACNM in 1981; now thirty-five years later the ACNM must make a stance.[4] It may necessitate putting concerns about academics, professionalism, and competition for delivery space aside, and collectively midwives must recognize that they are most effective before and during pregnancy. The evidence is indisputable: midwives excel at communication and education, and in the recognition of a woman's broader needs based on her social situation and culture. Moreover, midwifery increases access to health care in populations identified as high risk.[5] For a century or more, early and consistent prenatal care has been accepted as the key to lowering maternal and infant mortality and midwives are unrivaled at facilitating women's entry into macro-level care, but midwifery must be integral to the larger system lest we return to a care model that was proven to be deficient.

Beyond putting their own house in order, the leadership of the American College of Nurse-Midwives must ally with the medical establishment and policy makers to bring about positive change at the national level. Progress is being made to improve interprofessional understanding, and some mutual training programs are being initiated; the value of collaboration versus competition is finally being emphasized through initiatives such as the Alliance on Innovation for Maternal Health (AIM). Encouragingly, the American Congress of Obstetrics and Gynecology and the ACNM have joined forces to express their deep support of the Improving Access to Maternity Care Act. A larger presence at the federal level will help the ACNM achieve its goal of midwifery being "systemically recognized as a necessary part of any discussion related to women's health."[6]

Perhaps bringing most hope for the future of midwifery, though, is the recent US Midwifery Education, Regulation, and Association negotiations, and the delayed but eventual inclusion of ICTC. It was agreed that the education and licensing of all midwives should be raised in accordance with the International Confederation of Midwives standards and competencies, and for the first time, common ground was found on a collective philosophy of midwifery. Historically, the lack of standardization across the profession has been of great concern to physicians, but bringing particular optimism for the future is the fact that the 2014 president of the ACOG attended the negotiations and expressed support for the agreement, thus allowing for the prospect of midwifery to become more fully integrated into mainstream maternity care.[7] Signaling a new era the ACOG president declared: "This is a prime opportunity to not just collaborate with midwives, but also to learn from them."[8]

This new sense of solidarity between midwives of all backgrounds will not only foster more respect from physicians, but it brings with it an important opportunity to alter the American public's perception of midwifery. Because the term midwife has no standardized meaning in the United States, there is, and always has been, a good deal of misconception and confusion about the role. Through social media and public image campaigns, the ACNM is working hard to change the face of midwifery to bring it more in line with reality; the US MERA agreement will go far toward facilitating this shift. The president of the ACNM, Ginger Breedlove, hopes that the word midwife will soon be synonymous with someone who is a qualified and essential part of the health-care team.[9]

Change takes time, but is often accelerated by need and today, as was the case in the early twentieth century, American maternity care needs to be reevaluated so as to eliminate disparity and lower mortality for all women and infants. Revisiting the balancing scale analogy, the last one hundred years of African American maternity care has exhibited a shift from a predominance of micro care—traditional, empirical knowledge imparted by familiar, trusted practitioners at a community level—to being entirely weighted toward macro care, a highly technical care provided in a modern but distant facility, staffed by professionals that are far removed socially and culturally from their patients. History has shown that in this model, one type of care is sacrificed for the other to the detriment of the woman; racial disparities show the deficiency of the system. Ideally, an African American woman in a high-risk pregnancy as a result of chronic disease or poverty-related issues should not have to sacrifice the benefit of micro-level care in order to receive the macro care she certainly requires. In a better model, she would be fully supported by a network of properly credentialed community health workers (doulas, childbirth educators) that would ensure her full integration into early and regular prenatal care from midwives and physicians. Moving forward, one suggestion to take from this historical perspective would be to visualize the components of modern maternity care not as a balancing scale, but as onion layers, layers of micro and macro care building upon each other, enhancing each other, and supporting the patient as her needs demand. A woman identified as high risk will certainly be under the care of an obstetrician with access to state-of-the-art technology, but she is in no less need of culturally appropriate support, effective education on her medical condition, or the continuity of care that fosters a relationship of trust and respect; midwifery or at least elements of the midwifery model must enhance medicine. As someone who studies American maternity care, Dr. Eugene Declercq supports the adage, "Every mother deserves a midwife, and some need an obstetrician, too."[10]

Widening the focus away from the individual, groups like ICTC are leading the vanguard in high-risk, low-income communities to renew a legacy of midwifery, but without macro support in terms of integration and funding by state and federal agencies, they will fail. As Dr. J. Edward Hill pleaded in his state of American medicine address, activism at the local level is key, but leadership from the structural organizations of medicine and politics is essential for success in all medical specialties. He expressed disappointment in what he perceives as a lack of commitment from his profession, without which substantial change is unlikely.[11] Similarly, Dr. Thomas Boulware cautioned against the failure of the medical system to address modern challenges to the specialty of obstetrics, such as malpractice lawsuits and an overdependence on testing and technology. In the late 1980s he predicted the withdrawal of services and the subsequent creation of maternity care "deserts" in poor, rural areas. For Boulware, who believed that implicit in the Hippocratic Oath was an obligation to the poor, simply opting out of serving needy communities was anathema, and would result in a return to unsupervised, unsupported midwifery, thus turning back the clock on maternity care.[12]

The centrality of community to health care is being explored in other branches of medicine. An innovative study into hypertension in African American men found that the customers of a barbershop who had their blood pressure regularly checked by the barber were nine times more likely to seek treatment from a physician after encouragement from the barber than men who were simply given educational literature on hypertension.[13] Just as licensed midwives facilitated access to prenatal clinics in the mid-decades of the twentieth century, the consistent and familiar figure of the barber is bridging the gap between community and physician. (As a matter of fact, using barbers as an access point to black communities is not new; in 1933 they were identified as being ideally positioned as transmitters of public health information.)

Without the racial constraints of the Jim Crow era, a community-based foundation to well-being so well demonstrated by lay midwives may solve some of our current maternity care dilemmas. In describing his Mississippi Delta community that was plagued with high infant mortality rates, Dr. J. Edward Hill was adamant about forcing change: "We went to work with the state health department. We got donations from churches and from the March of Dimes, hired certified nurse-midwives, and developed a very strict protocol under which they acted. We trained women with not even a high school diploma to do home visiting including prenatal, perinatal, and postnatal visits. We educated and communicated, and in short order, infant mortality rates dropped below the national average."[14] This success story is not an example of a segregated African American community collaborating to meet its maternity care needs in the absence of science and modernity; this community mobilized in the 1970s, after Hill-Burton had populated the South with hospital beds, after the Civil Rights Act had desegregated medicine, and after lay midwifery had virtually been eliminated. Dr. Hill was galvanized into action when a woman came dangerously close to dying because of little access to basic medical care. The narrowly averted tragedy happened on July 20, 1969, the day Neil Armstrong took his giant leap for mankind. Fifty years after the moon landing and the expansion of science into all manner of unfathomable fields of inquiry, it is time to consider that increasing technology might not hold all the answers for maternity care and some less expensive, human intensive approaches may be more beneficial. It seems we have little to lose by turning to history to explore models of care that may have been discarded a little too easily in the name of progress.

NOTES

INTRODUCTION

1. Onnie Lee Logan as told to Katherine Clark, *Motherwit: An Alabama Midwife's Story* (New York: E. P. Dutton, 1989), ix.

2. Susan L. Smith, *Sick and Tired of Being Sick and Tired: Black Women's Health Activism in America, 1890–1950* (Philadelphia: University of Pennsylvania Press, 1995), 119.

3. Jesse Chambers, "Screening of 'Miss Margaret' Documentary in Eutaw," *Birmingham Weekly*, May 1, 2009. Eutaw, Alabama, is in Greene County, one of the ten counties in Alabama's Black Belt.

4. Southern Rural Black Women's Initiative, "Unequal Lives: The State of Black Women and Families in the Rural South," http://srbwi.org/index.php?/news (accessed August 28, 2017).

5. Dina Fine Maron, "Has Maternal Mortality Really Doubled in the U.S.?" *Scientific American*, June 8, 2015, http://www.scientificamerican.com/article/has-maternal -mortality-really-doubled-in-the-u-s/. The statement about the rising maternal mortality rate has been widely published in the mainstream media (e.g., *Atlantic Monthly*, *Economist*, CNN). However, Fine reports that it is less a sharp increase and more a result of better data collection of previously misclassified deaths.

6. US Department of Health and Human Services, Health Resources and Services Administration, Maternal and Child Health Bureau, *Child Health USA 2013* (Rockville, MD: US Department of Health and Human Services, 2013); "Deadly Delivery: The Maternity Health Care Crisis in the USA" (London: Amnesty International Secretariat, 2010), 1; Kelly Wallace, "Why Is the Maternal Mortality Rate Going up in the United States?" http://www.cnn.com/2015/12/01/health/maternal-mortality-rate-u-s-increasing -why/ (accessed December 11, 2015).

7. Jill Shatzen Kerr, *Burgess Leads Bipartisan Group in Introducing Bill to Improve Access to Maternity Care*, http://burgess.house.gov/news/documentsingle .aspx?DocumentID=397497 (accessed July 23, 2017). There were 1,163 first-year OB/ GYN residents in 1979 and 1,221 in 2014.

8. Eugene Declercq's figures quoted in American College Nurse-Midwives, *Improving Access to Maternity Care Act of 2015 (H.R. 1209/S.628)*, http://www.midwife.org/acnm/files/ccLibraryFiles/Filename/000000005035/MaternityShortageAreaLegislationTPs.pdf (accessed August 30, 2017).

9. Jamie Santa Cruz, "Call the Midwife," *Atlantic*, June 12, 2015, http://www.theatlantic.com/health/archive/2015/06/midwives-are-making-a-comeback/395456/ (accessed August 29, 2017).

10. J. Edward Hill, *The State of American Medicine*, Speech at The Denver Forum, October 25, 2006, http://www.thedenverforum.com/recent-speeches/the-state-of-american-medicine/ (accessed June 23, 2017).

11. Emilie M. Townes, *Breaking the Fine Rain of Death: African American Health Issues and a Womanist Ethic of Care* (New York: Continuum, 1998), 152.

12. Collins O. Airhihenbuwa and Leandris Liburd, "Eliminating Health Disparities in the African American Population: The Interface of Culture, Gender, and Power," *Education and Behavior* 33, no. 4 (August 2006): 491–96.

13. Melanie Beals Goan, *Mary Breckinridge: The Frontier Nursing Service and Rural Health in Appalachia* (Chapel Hill: University of North Carolina Press, 2008), 74.

14. Goan, *Mary Breckinridge*, 67.

15. Goan, *Mary Breckinridge*, 112.

16. Maria Milton, "Milton Memorial Birth Center: Continuing the Legacy of Black Midwifery in Florida with Maria Milton," *State of Black Midwifery Summit* (MP3), December 7, 2013, www.senadamarketing.com.

PART 1. MOTHERWIT: LAY MIDWIFERY

1. Logan, *Motherwit*, 59.

2. Sharla M. Fett, *Working Cures: Health, Healing, and Power on Southern Slave Plantations* (Chapel Hill: University of North Carolina Press, 2002), x.

CHAPTER 1: OUT OF SLAVERY

1. Fett, *Working Cures*, 199; Helen Varney Burst and Joyce Beebe Thompson, *A History of Midwifery in the United States* (New York: Springer Publishing Company, 2015), 10.

2. Marie Jenkins Schwartz, *Birthing a Slave; Motherhood and Medicine in the Antebellum South* (Cambridge, MA: Harvard University Press, 2009), 4.

3. Todd L. Savitt, *Race and Medicine in Nineteenth- and Early Twentieth-Century America* (Kent, OH: Kent State University Press, 2007), 61.

4. Steven M. Stowe, *Doctoring the South: Southern Physicians and Everyday Medicine in the Mid-Nineteenth Century* (Chapel Hill: University of North Carolina Press, 2004), 216.

5. Stowe, *Doctoring the South*, 218.

6. Fett, *Working Cures*, 20.

7. Schwartz, *Birthing a Slave*, 13.

8. Savitt, *Race and Medicine*, 68.

9. Christopher Morris, *Becoming Southern: The Evolution of a Way of Life, Warren County and Vicksburg, Mississippi, 1770–1860* (New York: Oxford University Press, 1995), 70–72.

10. Savitt, *Race and Medicine*, 68.

11. Savitt, *Race and Medicine*, 68.

12. Schwartz, *Birthing a Slave*, 96.

13. Schwartz, *Birthing a Slave*, 98; Ergot is a naturally occurring substance used for centuries to induce uterine contractions so as to promote the expulsion of a fetus or placenta, or to control hemorrhage.

14. Margaret Charles Smith and Linda Janet Holmes, *Listen to Me Good: The Life Story of an Alabama Midwife* (Columbus: Ohio State University Press, 1996), 24.

15. Laurie A. Wilkie, *The Archaeology of Mothering: An African American Midwife's Tale* (New York: Routledge, 2003), 61–62.

16. Morris, *Becoming Southern*, 71.

17. Fett, *Working Cures*, 138.

18. Wilkie, *The Archaeology of Mothering*, 119–45.

19. Fett, *Working Cures*, 141.

20. Schwartz, *Birthing a Slave*, 148. An infant born "with a veil on its face" is a lay term for when the infant is delivered with the amniotic membranes over its face. Individuals born this way were thought to possess a heightened spiritual awareness, have an ability to foresee the future, or simply have good fortune. It is a cross-cultural superstition. The veil is also known as a caul.

21. "List of Negroes belonging to Charles Kerrison, Esq.," Dr. Elizabeth M. Bear Collection, series 1, box 1, folder 3, Avery Research Center, College of Charleston, Charleston, South Carolina (ARC).

22. Fett, *Working Cures*, 198–200.

23. Jim Downs, *Sick from Freedom: African American Illness and Suffering during the Civil War and Reconstruction* (New York: Oxford University Press, 2012), 170.

24. Downs, *Sick from Freedom*, 75.

25. Downs, *Sick from Freedom*, 68.

26. Downs, *Sick from Freedom*, 69.

27. Schwartz, *Birthing a Slave*, 315.

CHAPTER 2. CULTURAL MOTIFS PERSIST

1. Grace L. Meigs, *Maternal Mortality from All Conditions Connected with Childbirth in the United States and Certain Other Countries*, United States Department of Labor,

Children's Bureau Publication, No. 19 (Washington, DC: US Government Printing Office, 1917), in *The American Midwife Debate: A Sourcebook on Its Modern Origins*, ed. Judy Barrett Litoff (New York: Greenwood Press, 1986), 61. There were a reported 15.2 deaths per 100,000 in the white population, 26.1 deaths per 100,000 in the black population. Norway and Sweden had the lowest rates; England, Ireland, and Japan had decreasing rates.

2. Litoff, *The American Midwife Debate*, 6.

3. W. C. Gewin, "Careless and Unscientific Midwifery with Special References to Some Features of the Work of Midwives," *Alabama Medical Journal*, Series 4, Vol. 11 (1905–6): 632, Reynolds-Finley Historical Library (RFHL), University of Alabama, Birmingham. The pioneer of aseptic technique was Ignaz Semmelweis, a Hungarian physician. In 1847 he observed that the incidence of puerperal fever was drastically reduced by the use of hand disinfection by doctors in his obstetric clinic. However, it was only after Louis Pasteur developed the germ theory of disease in the mid-1860s that Semmelweis's discovery was widely accepted.

4. Joseph B. De Lee, "Progress Toward Ideal Obstetrics," *Transactions of the American Association for the Study and Prevention of Infant Mortality* 6 (1915), 114–23, in *The American Midwife Debate: A Sourcebook on Its Modern Origins*, ed. Judy Barrett Litoff (New York: Greenwood Press, 1986), 102.

5. Diana Scully, "From Natural to Surgical Event," in *The American Way of Birth*, ed. Pamela S. Eakins (Philadelphia: Temple University Press, 1986), 47–59; Margarete Sandelowski, *Pain, Pleasure, and American Childbirth: From the Twilight Sleep to the Read Method, 1914–1960* (Westport, CT: Greenwood Press, 1984), 3–10.

6. Nancy Schrom Dye, "The Medicalization of Birth," in *The American Way of Birth*, ed. Pamela S. Eakins (Philadelphia: Temple University Press, 1986), 21–46; Judy Barrett Litoff, ed., *The American Midwife Debate: A Sourcebook on Its Modern Origins* (New York: Greenwood Press, 1986), 10.

7. Dye, "The Medicalization of Birth," 41, 42.

8. James C. Cobb, *The Most Southern Place on Earth: The Mississippi Delta and the Roots of Regional Identity* (Oxford: Oxford University Press, 1992), 264–65.

9. Smith and Holmes, *Listen to Me Good*, 86.

10. Thomas J. Ward Jr., *Black Physicians in the Jim Crow South* (Fayetteville: University of Arkansas Press, 2003), 103.

11. Sheila P. Davis and Cora Ingram, "Empowered Caretakers: A Historical Perspective on the Roles of Granny Midwives in Rural Alabama," in *Wings of Gauze: Women of Color and the Experience of Health and Illness*, ed. Barbara Blair and Susan E. Cayleff (Detroit: Wayne State University Press, 1993), 195; Wilkie, *The Archaeology of Mothering*, 142.

12. Logan, *Motherwit*, 50.

13. Claudine Curry Smith and Mildred H. B. Roberson, *My Bag Was Always Packed: The Life and Times of a Virginia Midwife* (Bloomington, IN: 1st Books Library, 2003), 122.

14. Logan, *Motherwit*, 48.

15. Linda Janet Holmes, "Louvenia Taylor Benjamin, Southern Lay Midwife: An Interview," *Sage* 2, no. 2 (Fall 1985): 52, http://www.proquest.com.

16. Smith and Holmes, *Listen to Me Good*, 71.

17. Smith and Holmes, *Listen to Me Good*, 23–30.

18. Logan, *Motherwit*, 89.

19. Smith and Holmes, *Listen to Me Good*, 85.

20. Judy Barrett Litoff, *American Midwives: 1860 to the Present* (New York: Greenwood Press, 1978), 32.

21. Logan, *Motherwit*, 88.

22. Logan, *Motherwit*, 89.

23. Davis, "Empowered Caretakers," 192.

24. Molly Dougherty, "Southern Midwives as Spiritual Specialists," *Women in Ritual and Symbolic Roles*, ed. Judith Hoch-Smith and Anita Spring (New York: Plenum Press, 1978), 153.

25. Holmes, "Louvenia Taylor Benjamin," 54.

26. Karen Kruse Thomas, *Deluxe Jim Crow: Civil Rights and American Health Policy, 1935–1954* (Athens: University of Georgia Press, 2011), 83.

27. Logan, *Motherwit*, 53.

28. Logan, *Motherwit*, 68.

29. Smith and Holmes, *Listen to Me Good*, 63.

30. Logan, *Motherwit*, 11–21.

31. Wendy Bovard and Gladys Milton, *Why Not Me? The Story of Gladys Milton, Midwife* (Summertown: The Book Publishing Company, 1993), 23.

32. Marie Campbell, *Folks Do Get Born* (New York: Rinehart, 1946), 82.

33. Mary B. Hilliard, interviewed by Daisy M. Greene, October 19, 1977, Washington County Library System Oral History Project, Mississippi Department of Archives and History.

34. Smith and Holmes, *Listen to Me Good*, 75.

35. Campbell, *Folks Do Get Born*, 46.

36. Smith and Holmes, *Listen to Me Good*, 76.

37. "Leflore Midwife Fails on Fee, Takes Baby," *Jackson Daily News*, November 8, 1939, series 2036, box 8416, folder County Files Amite-Grenada, 1939–1951, MDAH.

38. Smith and Roberson, *My Bag Was Always Packed*, 88.

CHAPTER 3. LICENSING AND THE "NEW LAWS"

1. Meigs, *Maternal Mortality*, 63.

2. Grace Abbott, "Federal Aid for the Protection of Maternity and Infancy," *American Journal of Public Health* 12, no. 9 (September 1922): 737–42.

3. Mississippi State Board of Health, "Midwife Supervision," Midwife Program Files and Photographs—Public Health Nursing Division, 1911–1976, box 8416, series 2036, folder Midwife Supervision (1938?), MDAH.

4. Felix J. Underwood, "The Development of Midwifery in Mississippi," *Southern Medical Journal* 19, no. 9 (1926): 683, Collection MC53, Folder 4.63. UAB Archives; E. R. Hardin, "The Midwife Problem," *Southern Medical Journal* 18 (May 1925), in *The American Midwife Debate: A Sourcebook on Its Modern Origins*, ed. Judy Barrett Litoff (New York: Greenwood Press, 1986), 147.

5. Mississippi State Board of Health, "Policies Regarding Midwife Supervision," Mississippi State Board of Health, 1948, Midwife Program Files and Photographs—Public Health Nursing Division, 1911–1976, 8416, series 2036, box 8416, folder Midwife Supervision, MDAH.

6. Alabama State Department of Health, "Midwife Record," 1942, series 1, box 1, folder 2, Dr. Elizabeth M. Bear Collection, ARC; Mississippi State Board of Health, *Lesson Outlines for Teaching Midwives*, 1939, 2, MDAH.

7. E. R. Hardin, "The Midwife Problem," *Southern Medical Journal* 18 (May 1925): 347–50, in *The American Midwife Debate: A Sourcebook on Its Modern Origins*, ed. Judy Barrett Litoff (New York: Greenwood Press, 1986), 148.

8. Mississippi State Board of Health, "The Relation of the Midwife to the State Board of Health," 1931, Midwife Program Files and Photographs—Public Health Nursing Division, 1911–1976, series 2036, box 8416, folder The Relation of the Midwife to the State Board of Health, MDAH.

9. Susan L. Smith, *Sick and Tired*, 118.

10. Mississippi State Board of Health, "The Relation of the Midwife to the State Board of Health," 1931.

11. Katherine Hagquist, "Report on the Midwifery Survey in Texas," Bureau of Child Hygiene, Texas State Board of Health, 1924, in *The American Midwife Debate: A Sourcebook on Its Modern Origins*, ed. Judy Barrett Litoff (New York: Greenwood Press, 1986), 75.

12. E. R. Hardin, "The Midwife Problem," *Southern Medical Journal* 18 (May 1925): 347–50, in *The American Midwife Debate: A Sourcebook on Its Modern Origins*, ed. Judy Barrett Litoff (New York: Greenwood Press, 1986), 146.

13. Smith and Holmes, *Listen to Me Good*, 65.

14. Smith, *Sick and Tired*, 124.

15. Mississippi State Board of Health, "The Relation of the Midwife to the State Board of Health," 1931, MDAH.

16. Hagquist, "Report on the Midwifery Survey in Texas," 71.

17. Molly Ladd-Taylor, "Grannies and Spinsters: Midwife Education under the Sheppard-Towner Act," *Journal of Social History* 22, no. 2 (Winter 1988): 267.

18. Mississippi State Board of Health, *Manual for Midwives*, 1931, 7; Mississippi State Board of Health, *Lesson Outlines for Teaching Midwives*, 1939; Mississippi State Board

of Health, "The Relation of the Midwife to the State Board of Health," 1938(?), Midwife Program Files and Photographs—Public Health Nursing Division, 1911–1976, series 2036, box 8416, folder The Relation of the Midwife to the State Board of Health, MDAH.

19. South Carolina State Board of Health, *Lessons for Midwives*, Revised 1970, Dr. Elizabeth M. Bear Collection, Folder 2, Nurse-Midwife Education, 1941–1970, ARC.

20. Mississippi State Board of Health, "The Relation of the Midwife to the State Board of Health," 1938(?).

21. James H. Ferguson, "Mississippi Midwives," *Journal of the History of Medicine* (Winter 1950): 89; Mississippi State Board of Health, "Teaching Guide—Midwife Supervision," Chapter 3, Midwife Clubs, MDAH; Mississippi State Board of Health, *Manual for Midwives*, 1931.

22. Mississippi State Board of Health, "Policies Regarding Midwife Supervision," 1948, Midwife Program Files and Photographs—Public Health Nursing Division, 1911–1976, series 2036, box 8416, folder Midwife Supervision, MDAH.

23. Campbell, *Folks Do Get Born*, 42.

24. Campbell, *Folks Do Get Born*, 43.

25. Mississippi State Board of Health, "The Relation of the Midwife to the State Board of Health," 1938(?).

CHAPTER 4. IMPLEMENTING THE CHANGES

1. Lillie Bell Hill, Annual Report for the Lee County Midwives Club, 1937, Midwife Program Files and Photographs—Public Health Nursing Division, 1911–1976, series 2036, box 8416, folder Relation of Midwife to the State Board of Health, MDAH.

2. Logan, *Motherwit*, 137.

3. Mississippi State Board of Health, *Manual for Midwives*, 1931, 15.

4. Alabama State Department of Public Health, *The Alabama Midwife: Her Book* (Montgomery: Alabama State Department of Public Health, 1956), 14–15, original in possession of Arrol Sheehan, Alabama Department of Public Health, Montgomery, Alabama; Virginia State Department of Health, *Midwife's Manual*, 15, in Smith and Roberson, *My Bag Was Always Packed*, 159.

5. Logan, *Motherwit*, 137.

6. Alabama State Department of Public Health, *The Alabama Midwife: Her Book*, 11; South Carolina State Board of Health, *Lessons for Midwives*, 24.

7. Smith and Roberson, *My Bag Was Always Packed*, 159; Mississippi State Board of Health, *Manual for Midwives*, 1931, 15–24.

8. Mississippi State Board of Health, *Lesson Outlines for Teaching Midwives*, 1939, 7.

9. Mississippi State Board of Health, "Midwife Supervision," 1938(?), Midwife Program Files and Photographs—Public Health Nursing Division, 1911–1976, series 2036, box 8416, folder The Relationship of the Midwife to the State Board of Health, MDAH; Smith, *Sick*

and Tired, 145–46; "Midwives and Health Work," newspaper article, September 30, 1933, Midwife Program Files and Photographs—Public Health Nursing Division, 1911–1976, series 2036, box 8416, folder Letters describing delivery room displays, MDAH.

10. Smith and Holmes, *Listen to Me Good*, 75.

11. Smith and Holmes, *Listen to Me Good*, 88.

12. Logan, *Motherwit*, 93–94.

13. Davis, "Empowered Caretakers," 195.

14. Logan, *Motherwit*, 93; Smith and Roberson, *My Bag Was Always Packed*, 56; Smith and Holmes, *Listen to Me Good*, 88; Bovard and Milton, *Why Not Me?* 47.

15. Smith and Roberson, *My Bag Was Always Packed*, 66.

16. Medical Association of the State of Alabama, *Transactions of the Medical Association of the State of Alabama* (Montgomery: Medical Association of the State of Alabama, 1940), 13, Reynolds-Finley Historical Library (RFHL), University of Alabama at Birmingham.

17. George C. Stoney, *All My Babies: A Midwife's Own Story*, Film directed by George C. Stoney (Atlanta: Georgia Department of Public Health, 1953).

18. Logan, *Motherwit*, 136; Alabama State Department of Health, A General Daily Guide During Normal Pregnancy (1958), Bureau of Maternal and Child Health, LPR 315, Box 2, Folder 8, Datcher Family Collection (DFC), Alabama Department of Archives and History (ADAH), Montgomery, Alabama.

19. Mississippi State Board of Health, "The Relationship of the Midwife to the State Board of Health," 1931.

20. Carey V. Stabler, "The History of Alabama Public Health System" (PhD diss., Duke University, 1944), 262.

21. Medical Association of the State of Alabama (MASA), *Transactions*, 1950, 4.

22. MASA, *Transactions*, 1935, 10.

23. Smith and Holmes, *Listen to Me Good*, 35.

24. Smith and Holmes, *Listen to Me Good*, 49.

25. Logan, *Motherwit*, 130.

26. Gertrude Jacinta Fraser, *African American Midwifery in the South: Dialogues of Birth, Race, and Memory* (Cambridge, MA: Harvard University Press), ch. 6; Stabler, "Alabama Public Health System," 262.

27. Harriet A. Washington, *Medical Apartheid: The Dark History of Medical Experimentation on Black Americans from Colonial Times to the Present* (New York: Anchor Books, 2006), 5

28. Logan, *Motherwit*, 102.

29. Washington, *Medical Apartheid*, 204; Dr. Helen Barnes, personal interview with Jenny Luke, Jackson, Mississippi, December 29, 2012.

30. Smith and Holmes, *Listen to Me Good*, 83.

31. Logan, *Motherwit*, 65.

32. Ladd-Taylor, "Grannies and Spinsters," 268; "Forrest County's Midwives Do Their Job Well," August 23, 1950, Midwife Program Files and Photographs—Public Health Nursing Division, 1911–1976, series 2036, box 8416, folder County Files, Amite-Grenada, 1939–1951, MDAH.

33. Smith and Holmes, *Listen to Me Good*, 99.

34. South Carolina State Board of Health, *Lessons for Midwives*, 7.

35. Alabama Department of Health, *The Alabama Midwife: Her Book*, 5–7.

36. Anita M. Jones, RN, *Manual for Teaching Midwives* (Washington, DC: United States Department of Labor, Children's Bureau, 1941), 6, RFHL.

37. Ladd-Taylor, "Grannies and Spinsters," 267.

38. Campbell, *Folks Do Get Born*, 30.

39. Linda Janet Holmes, "African American Midwives in the South," in *The American Way of Birth*, ed. Pamela S. Eakins (Philadelphia: Temple University Press, 1986), 277.

40. Detrice G. Barry and Joyceen S. Boyle, "An Ethnohistory of a Granny Midwife," *Journal of Transcultural Nursing* 8, no. 1 (July–December 1996): 16.

41. Logan, *Motherwit*, 95; Smith and Roberson, *My Bag Was Always Packed*, 56; Smith, *Sick and Tired*, 120; Bovard and Milton, *Why Not Me?* 47; Campbell, *Folks Do Get Born*, 87.

42. Sandelowski, *Pain, Pleasure, and American Childbirth*, 68–70.

43. Smith and Roberson, *My Bag Was Always Packed*, 65.

44. Debra Anne Susie, *The Way of Our Grandmothers: A Cultural View of Twentieth-Century Midwifery in Florida* (Athens: University of Georgia Press, 1988), 21.

45. Holmes, "Louvenia Taylor Benjamin," 51.

46. Campbell, *Folks Do Get Born*, 84.

CHAPTER 5. WORKING WITH THE STATE

1. Midwife Report, Estelle W. Christian to Miss Viola M. Jones, October 5, 1939, Midwife Program Files and Photographs—Public Health Nursing Division, 1911–1976, series 2036, box 8416, folder County Files Armite—Grenada, 1939–1951, MDAH.

2. Laura Blackburn, "The Midwife as an Ally," *American Journal of Nursing* 42, no. 1 (January 1942): 57.

3. Mississippi State Board of Health, "The Relationship of the Midwife to the State Board of Health," 1938(?) (excerpts from Midwife Club Reports), MDAH.

4. Mississippi State Board of Health, "The Relationship of the Midwife to the State Board of Health," 1931.

5. Logan, *Motherwit*, 98–99.

6. Logan, *Motherwit*, 100.

7. MASA, *Transactions*, 1933, 10, RFHL; MASA, *Transactions*, 1937, 12, RFHL. The Maternal and Infant Welfare Committee reports are from 1933 to 1956.

8. Fraser, *African American Midwifery in the South*, 71–77.

9. Alabama State Department of Public Health, *The Alabama Midwife: Her Book*, 59–60; South Carolina State Board of Health, *Lessons for Midwives*, 72–78; Smith and Roberson, *My Bag Was Always Packed*, 155–62. A copy of the midwives' manual is included as an appendix to the book.

10. Anita M. Jones, *Manual for Teaching Midwives* (Washington, DC: US Government Printing Office, 1941), 135, RFHL.

11. Patricia Evridge Hill, "Dr. Hilla Sheriff: Caught Between Science and the State at the South Carolina Midwife Training Institutes," in *South Carolina Women: Their Lives and Times, Volume 3*, ed. Marjorie Julian Spruill, Valinda W. Littlefield, and Joan Marie Johnson (Athens: University of Georgia Press, 2012), 90.

12. Hill, "Dr. Hilla Sheriff."

CHAPTER 6. WORKING WITH PHYSICIANS

1. Logan, *Motherwit*, 59.

2. Smith and Holmes, *Listen to Me Good*, 104.

3. Smith and Roberson, *May Bag Was Always Packed*, 96.

4. Bovard and Milton, *Why Not Me?* 77.

5. Bovard and Milton, *Why Not Me?* 36.

6. Smith and Roberson, *My Bag Was Always Packed*, 60.

7. Smith, *Sick and Tired*, 140.

8. Logan, *Motherwit*, 166.

9. Felix J. Underwood, "The Development of Midwifery in Mississippi," 683.

10. Mississippi State Board of Health, "The Relationship of the Midwife to the State Board of Health," 1931, MDAH.

11. Deborah Shelton Pinkney, "Onnie's Children; Mobile County's Last Lay Midwife, Onnie Lee Logan, Delivered Babies and Goodwill," *American Medical News* 33, no. 15 (April 20, 1990). Dr. J. M. Robinson's comments about Onnie Lee Logan.

12. Mississippi State Board of Health, "The Relationship of the Midwife to the State Board of Health," 1931, MDAH.

13. Smith and Holmes, *Listen to Me Good*, 88; Margaret Charles Smith, interview by Ina Gaskin May, *Birth Gazette* 13, no. 1 (Winter 1996): 6.

14. Smith and Roberson, *My Bag Was Always Packed*, 120.

15. Holmes, "Louvenia Taylor Benjamin," 54.

PART 2. ASAFETIDA TO AUREOMYCIN: AFRICAN AMERICAN NURSE-MIDWIVES

1. W. Eugene Smith, "Nurse Midwife: Maude Callen Eases the Pain of Birth, Life and Death," *Life*, December 3, 1951, 134–45.

2. Smith, "Nurse Midwife," 135.

CHAPTER 7. ESTABLISHING THE PROFESSIONAL NURSE-MIDWIFE

1. De Lee, "Progress Toward Ideal Obstetrics," in Litoff, *The American Midwife Debate*, 102.

2. *Good Housekeeping* (1926), 88: 270, quoted in Judith Walzer Leavitt, "Joseph B. De Lee and the Practice of Preventive Obstetrics," *American Journal of Public Health* 78, no. 10 (1988): 1353–61.

3. De Lee, "Progress Toward Ideal Obstetrics," 105.

4. Maternity Center Association, *Twenty Years of Nurse-Midwifery, 1933–1953* (New York: Maternity Center Association, 1955), 12.

5. Maternity Center Association, *Twenty Years of Nurse-Midwifery*, 13.

6. Maternity Center Association, *Twenty Years of Nurse-Midwifery*, 14.

7. An example of the "necessary evil" argument can be found in J. Clifton Edgar, "The Education, Licensing, and Supervision of the Midwife," *American Journal of Obstetrics and the Diseases of Women and Children* 73 (March 1916): 385–98, in Litoff, *The American Midwife Debate*, 129–43.

8. Carolyn Conant Van Blarcom, "Midwives in America," *American Journal of Public Health* 4 (March 1914): 197–207, in Litoff, *The American Midwife Debate*, 174.

9. Abraham Jacobi, "The Best Means of Combating Infant Mortality," *Journal of the American Medical Association* 58 (June 1912): 1735–44, in Litoff, *The American Midwife Debate*, 177–99.

10. Laura Ettinger, *Nurse-Midwifery: The Birth of a New Profession* (Columbus: Ohio State University Press, 2006), 81; Varney Burst and Thompson, *A History of Midwifery in the United States*, 78.

11. Maternity Center Association, *Twenty Years of Nurse-Midwifery*, 18, 19; Varney Burst and Thompson, *A History of Midwifery in the United States*, 107.

12. Maternity Center Association, *Twenty Years of Nurse-Midwifery*, 18. The puerperium is the period of time following delivery during which the reproductive organs return to their normal state, usually considered to be six weeks.

13. Ettinger, *Nurse-Midwifery*, 85.

14. Maternity Center Association, *Twenty Years of Nurse-Midwifery*, 25–26; Ettinger, *Nurse-Midwifery*, 88.

15. Maternity Center Association, *Twenty Years of Nurse-Midwifery*, 115–24.

16. Maternity Center Association, *Twenty Years of Nurse-Midwifery*, 28.

17. H. M. Wallace, MD, "Trends in Maternal and Perinatal Mortality in New York City," *Journal of American Medical Association* (June 1954): 717, qtd. in Maternity Center Association, *Twenty Years of Nurse-Midwifery*, 29.

18. Maternity Center Association, *Twenty Years of Nurse-Midwifery*, 36.

19. Varney Burst and Thompson, *A History of Midwifery in the United States*, 89–95.

20. Hill, "Dr. Hilla Sheriff," 84.

21. Hill, "Dr. Hilla Sheriff," 85.

22. Charles H. Peckham, "The Essentials of Adequate Maternal Care in Rural Areas," *The Child* 5 (November 1939): 123, qtd. in Maternity Center Association, *Twenty Years of Nurse-Midwifery*, 56.

23. Francis Rothert, *Maternal Mortality in Fifteen States* (Washington, DC: Department of Labor, Children's Bureau Publication Number 223, 1934), 63.

24. MASA, *Transactions*, 1940, 12, RFHL.

25. MASA, *Transactions*, 1950, 4, RFHL.

CHAPTER 8. AFRICAN AMERICAN NURSE-MIDWIVES

1. Ettinger, *Nurse-Midwifery*, 149; Varney Burst and Thompson, *A History of Midwifery in the United States*, 114.

2. Maternity Center Association, *Twenty Years of Nurse-Midwifery*, 58–59; Varney Burst and Thompson, *A History of Midwifery in the United States*, 112–13.

3. Letter from Constance Manning to Claudia M. Durham, August 2, 1945, Dr. Elizabeth M. Bear Collection, series 1, box 1, folder 2, ARC.

4. Varney Burst and Thompson, *A History of Midwifery in the United States*, 113.

5. Maternity Center Association, *Twenty Years of Nurse-Midwifery*, 61.

6. Lucinda Canty, "The Graduates of the Tuskegee School of Nurse-Midwifery" (Master's thesis, Yale University, 1994).

7. Maternity Center Association, *Twenty Years of Nurse-Midwifery*, table 1, 24.

8. Darlene Clark Hine, *Black Women in White: Racial Conflict and Cooperation in the Nursing Profession, 1890–1950* (Bloomington: Indiana University Press, 1989), 65.

9. Tuskegee Institute, Alabama, "Bulletin of the Tuskegee School of Nurse-Midwifery, 1945," Dr. Elizabeth M. Bear Collection, series 1, box 1, folder 2, ARC.

10. Estelle G. Massey Riddle, "The Training and Placement of Negro Nurses," *Journal of Negro Education* 4 (1935): 42–48, in *Black Women in the Nursing Profession: A Documentary History*, ed. Darlene Clark Hine (New York: Garland Publishing, 1985), 91.

11. Canty, "Graduates of Tuskegee," 26–36; Hine, *Black Women in the Nursing Profession*, 89–95; Hine, *Black Women in White*, 63–84.

12. Canty, "Graduates of Tuskegee," 26–27.

13. Lucinda Canty, "Tuskegee School of Nurse-Midwifery" presentation at Hartford Hospital, docplayer.net/8953608-Tuskegee-school-of-nurse-midwidery-lucinda-canty-cnm-ms … (accessed July 7, 2017); Letter from Constance Manning Durrell to Betty (Dr. Elizabeth M. Bear), May 20, 1980, Dr. Elizabeth M. Bear Collection, series 1, box 1, folder 2, ARC.

14. Tuskegee Institute, Alabama, "Bulletin of the Tuskegee School of Nurse-Midwifery," 1945, ARC; Dorothy Deming, "The Negro Nurse in Public Health," *Journal of Negro Life* 15 (November 1937): 333–35, in Hine, *Black Women in the Nursing Profession*, 99.

15. Abie Roberts, "Nursing Education and Opportunities for the Colored Nurse," *Proceedings of the National Conference of Social Work* (Chicago: Chicago University Press, 1928), 183–85, in Hine, *Black Women in the Nursing Profession*, 62.

16. Boulware drafts (written as a history of Boulware in Birmingham), MC53, box 4, folder 15, UAB Archives.

17. Lucie Robertson Bridgforth, "The Politics of Public Health Reform: Felix J. Underwood and the Mississippi State Board of Health, 1924–58," *Public Historian* 6, no. 3 (Summer 1884): 12.

18. Darlene Clark Hine, "African American Women and Their Communities in the Twentieth Century," *Black Women, Gender, and Families* 1, no. 1 (Spring 2007): 15.

19. Dorothy Deming, "The Negro Nurse in Public Health," *Journal of Negro Life* 15 (November 1937): 333–35, in Hine, *Black Women in the Nursing Profession*, 99; Nina D. Gage and Alma C. Haupt, "Some Observations on Negro Nursing in the South," *Public Health Nursing* 24 (1932): 674–80, in Hine, *Black Women in the Nursing Profession*, 81–87.

20. John A. Kenney, "The First Graduating Class of the Tuskegee School of Midwifery," *Journal of the National Medical Association* 34, no. 3 (May 1942): 107.

21. Kenney, "The First Graduating Class of the Tuskegee School of Midwifery," 108.

22. Tuskegee Institute, *The Bulletin of the Tuskegee School of Nurse-Midwifery*, 8–10, ARC.

23. Tuskegee Institute, *The Bulletin of the Tuskegee School of Nurse-Midwifery*, 6, ARC; Letter from Constance Manning to Claudia M. Durham, August 2, 1945, Dr. Elizabeth M. Bear Collection, series 1, box 1, folder 2, ARC.

24. Deming, "The Negro Nurse in Public Health," 99.

25. M. O. Bousfield, "Reaching the Negro Community," *American Journal of Public Health* 24, no. 3 (March 1934): 211.

26. Stanley Rayfield, "A Study of Negro Public Health Nursing," *Public Health Nurse* (October 1930): 525–36, in. Hine, *Black Women in the Nursing Profession*, 71.

27. Kenney, "The First Graduating Class of the Tuskegee School of Midwifery," 109.

28. Hill, "Dr. Hilla Sheriff," 86.

29. W. Eugene Smith, "Nurse-Midwife: Maude Callen," 141.

30. Letter from Constance Manning Durrell to Betty (Dr. Elizabeth M. Bear), May 20, 1980, ARC.

31. W. Eugene Smith, "Nurse-Midwife: Maude Callen," 135.

32. Hill, "Dr. Hilla Sheriff," 89.

33. Jones, *Manual for Teaching Midwives*, vii.

34. Jones, *Manual for Teaching Midwives*, foreword by Margaret Murphy in amended copy for Alabama, VI-1.

35. Linda Janet Holmes, *Into the Light of Day: Reflections on the History of Midwives of Color within the American College of Nurse-Midwives* (Silver Spring, MD: American College of Nurse-Midwives, 2012), 19.

CHAPTER 9. THE APPLICATION OF NURSE-MIDWIVES

1. Pegge L. Bell, "'Making Do' with the Midwife: Arkansas's Mamie O. Hale," *Nursing History Review* 1 (1993): 159.

2. Hill, "Dr. Hilla Sheriff," 77. In South Carolina the maternal mortality rate fell from 540 per 10,000 live births in 1945 to 175 per 10,000 in 1957. The number of stillbirths per 1,000 fell from 47.4 to 27.1 between the same years.

3. Miscellaneous magazine articles on the Penn Center in Dr. Elizabeth M. Bear Collection, Penn Center, 1940–2006, series 2, box 1, folder 6, ARC.

4. Laura Blackburn, "The Midwife Problem in Rural Areas of the South," *The Trained Nurse and Hospital Review* (1939): 129.

5. Hill, "Dr. Hilla Sheriff," 87; Ferguson, "Mississippi Midwives," 89.

6. W. Eugene Smith, "Nurse-Midwife: Maude Callen," 145.

7. Hill, "Dr. Hilla Sheriff," 87.

8. Beatrice Mongeau, "The Granny Midwife: Changing Roles and Functions of a Folk Practitioner," *American Journal of Sociology* 66, no. 5 (March 1961): 497–505.

9. Jones, *Manual for Teaching Midwives*, 1–3.

10. Blackburn, "The Midwife Problem in Rural Areas of the South," 130.

11. Bell, "'Making Do' with the Midwife," 162.

12. Jones, *Manual for Teaching Midwives*, 64–75.

13. Jones, *Manual for Teaching Midwives*, 104.

14. Jones, *Manual for Teaching Midwives*, 120.

15. Smith and Holmes, *Listen to Me Good*, 96.

16. *Manual for Midwives, 1931*, Mississippi State Board of Health, 40, MDAH; Ferguson, "Mississippi Midwives," 92.

17. Hill, "Dr. Hilla Sheriff," 90.

18. W. Eugene Smith, "Nurse-Midwife: Maude Callen," 135.

19. Ettinger, *Nurse-Midwifery*, 151.

CHAPTER 10. PROBLEMS OF RACISM AND CHALLENGES TO PROFESSIONALISM

1. Ettinger, *Nurse-Midwifery*, 180. Please see chapter 13 for more about the American College of Nurse-Midwives.

2. Boulware Drafts (Written as a history of Boulware in Birmingham), MC 53, 4.15, UAB.

3. Estelle G. Massey, "Sources of Supply of Negro Health Personnel," *Journal of Negro Education* 6 (1937): 483–92, in Hine, *Black Women in the Nursing Profession*, 103–11; Canty, "Graduates of Tuskegee," 34.

4. Letters between Margaret W. Thomas and Margaret S. Vaughan, dated October 1943, Dr. Elizabeth M. Bear Collection, ARC. Mamie O. Hale is mentioned in the letter as a potential recruit.

5. Stanley Rayfield, "A Study of Negro Public Health Nursing," *Public Health Nurse* (October 1930): 525–36, in Hine, *Black Women in the Nursing Profession*, 71.

6. Letter from Constance Manning to Claudia M. Durham, August 2, 1945, Dr. Elizabeth M. Bear Collection, series 1, box 1, folder 2, ARC.

7. Medical Association of the State of Alabama, *Transactions of the Medical Association of the State of Alabama* (Montgomery: Medical Association of the State of Alabama, 1944), 29, MC 53, box 4, folder 3, University of Alabama at Birmingham Archives, Birmingham, Alabama.

8. Katherine Louise Dawley, "Leaving the Nest: Nurse-Midwifery in the United States, 1940–1980" (PhD diss., University of Pennsylvania, 2001), 79.

9. Maternity Center Association, *Twenty Years of Nurse-Midwifery*, 61.

10. Canty, "Graduates of Tuskegee," 34.

11. Ward Jr., *Black Physicians in the Jim Crow South*, 123.

12. Bruce Bellingham and Mary Pugh Mathis, "Race, Citizenship, and the Bio-ethics of the Maternalist Welfare State: 'Traditional' Midwifery in the American South under the Sheppard-Towner Act, 1921–29," *Social Politics* 1, no. 2 (1994): 158–59, 173, in Hill, "Dr. Hilla Sheriff," 84.

13. Edward J. Beardsley, *A History of Neglect: Health Care for Blacks and Mill Workers in the Twentieth-Century South* (Knoxville: University of Tennessee Press, 1987), 175–76.

14. Fraser, *African American Midwifery in the South*, 103.

15. Airhihenbuwa and Liburd, "Eliminating Health Disparities in the African American Population," 488–501.

PART 3. CHANGING ATTITUDES AND BETTER ACCESS

1. Fraser, *African American Midwifery in the South*, 134.

CHAPTER 11. OVERCOMING CHALLENGES

1. Beardsley, *A History of Neglect*, 34.

2. Ward Jr., *Black Physicians in the Jim Crow South*, 153.

3. Beardsley, *A History of Neglect*, 36.

4. Beardsley, *A History of Neglect*, 77.

5. Ward Jr., *Black Physicians in the Jim Crow South*, 3.

6. Beardsley, *A History of Neglect*, 78.

7. Ward Jr., *Black Physicians in the Jim Crow South*, 18.

8. Ward Jr., *Black Physicians in the Jim Crow South*, 37–39.

9. Douglas L. Conner with John F. Marszalek, *A Black Physician's Story: Bringing Hope in Mississippi* (Jackson: University Press of Mississippi, 1985), 67.

10. Conner with Marszalek, *A Black Physician's Story*, 68.

11. James T. Montgomery, MD, interviewed by Virginia Fisher, August 26, 1987, MC45 1.45, UAB.

12. Boulware Drafts (written as a history of Boulware in Birmingham), MC53, Folder 4.15, UAB.

13. James T. Montgomery, MD, interviewed by Virginia Fisher, August 26, 1987, MC45 1.45, UAB.

14. Vanessa Northington Gamble, *Making a Place for Ourselves: The Black Hospital Movement, 1920–1945* (Oxford: Oxford University Press, 1995), 29.

15. Michael M. Davis and Hugh H. Smythe, "Providing Adequate Health Service to Negroes," *Journal of Negro Education* 18, no. 3, The Health Status and Health Education of Negroes in the United States (Summer 1949): 310.

16. Ward Jr., *Black Physicians in the Jim Crow South*, 60.

17. Conner, *A Black Physician's Story*, 78.

18. Letter from Tinsley R. Harrison, MD to Mr. Brewer Dixon, May 7, 1951, MC 53, 4.35, UAB.

19. Conner, *A Black Physician's Story*, 75.

20. Conner, *A Black Physician's Story*, 82.

21. Conner, *A Black Physician's Story*, 77.

22. Dr. Helen Barnes, interview by Jenny Luke, Jackson, Mississippi, December 29, 2012.

23. Ward Jr., *Black Physicians in the Jim Crow South*, 187.

24. Gamble, *Making a Place for Ourselves*, 35–36; Beardsley, *A History of Neglect*, 82.

25. Karen Kruse Thomas, "The Hill-Burton Act and Civil Rights: Expanding Hospital Care for Black Southerners, 1939–1960," *Journal of Southern History* 72, no. 4 (November 2006): 826.

26. David T. Beito and Linda Royster Beito, "'Let Down Your Bucket Where You Are': The Afro-American Hospital and Black Health Care in Mississippi, 1924–1966," *Social Science History* 30, no. 4 (Winter 2006): 558.

27. Beardsley, *A History of Neglect*, 91.

28. Boulware Drafts (written as a history of Boulware in Birmingham), MC53, Folder 4.15, UAB.

29. Gamble, *Making a Place for Ourselves*, 56.

30. Edward H. Beardsley, "Desegregating Southern Medicine, 1945–1970," *International Social Science Review* 71, no. 1 & 2 (1996): 38.

31. Thomas, *Deluxe Jim Crow*; Beardsley, *A History of Neglect*, 178.

32. Forest E. Ludden, *The History of Public Health in Alabama (1941–1968)* (Montgomery: Alabama Department of Public Health, 1970), 92.

33. Ward Jr., *Black Physicians in the Jim Crow South*, 177.

34. Beardsley, "Desegregating Southern Medicine, 1945–1970," 43.

35. David Barton Smith, "The Politics of Racial Disparities: Desegregating the Hospitals in Jackson, Mississippi," *Milbank Quarterly* 83, no. 2 (2005): 258.

36. Ludden, *The History of Public Health in Alabama*, 94–96.

37. Kruse, *Deluxe Jim Crow*, 176–81; Beardsley, *A History of Neglect*, 156–85; Ward Jr., *Black Physicians in the Jim Crow South*, 187.

38. University of Alabama Board of Trustees, "A Chronological History of the University of Alabama at Birmingham and Its Predecessor Institutions and Organizations, 1831–," https://www.uab.edu/archives/chron.

39. Beardsley, "Desegregating Southern Medicine, 1945–1970," 50.

40. Beito and Beito, "'Let Down Your Bucket Where You Are,'" 564.

41. Walter H. Maddux, MD, "The Slossfield Health Center: An Example of Local Medical Service for Mothers and Children under the Public Health Auspices," *American Journal of Public Health* 31 (May 1941): 485.

42. T. M. Boulware, Elizabeth LaForge, and R. C. Stewart, "A Negro Demonstration Center for Maternal and Newborn Care in Alabama," *Southern Medical Journal* 36, no. 12 (December 1943), MC33 folder 1.5, UAB.

43. Thomas M. Boulware, MD, interviewed by Virginia Fisher, June 30, 1987, MC45, folder 1.17, UAB.

44. Boulware, LaForge, and Stewart, "A Negro Demonstration Center for Maternal and Newborn Care in Alabama," MC33 folder 1.5, UAB.

45. Boulware, LaForge, and Stewart, "A Negro Demonstration Center for Maternal and Newborn Care in Alabama," MC33 1.5, UAB; MASA, *Transactions*, 1943, RFHL; Boulware drafts, UAB.

46. Jennifer Nelson, "Healthcare Reconsidered: Forging Community Wellness among African Americans in the South," *Bulletin of the History of Medicine* 81, no. 3 (2007): 594–624.

47. Maddux, "The Slossfield Health Center," 485.

48. Nelson, "Healthcare Reconsidered," 603, 604.

49. Nelson, "Healthcare Reconsidered," 615.

50. Boulware drafts, UAB; MASA, *Transactions*, 1949, 41, UAB; Slossfield Health Center, 1940, MC53, box 4, folder 7, UAB.

51. Beardsley, *A History of Neglect*, 174.

52. Maternal Mortality in Alabama, 1952, MC29, box 2, folder 55, UAB.

CHAPTER 12. AFRICAN AMERICAN WOMEN TURN TO HOSPITAL BIRTH

1. Ferguson, "Mississippi Midwives," 89; Thomas, *Deluxe Jim Crow*, 60, 86; Beardsley, *A History of Neglect*, 277.

2. MASA, *Transactions*, 1935, 9, RFHL.

3. *A Report on the Five-Year Study of Maternal Mortality in Alabama, 1944–1948*, Committee on Maternal and Child Health of the Medical Association of the State of Alabama, MC29, Folder 2.55, UAB; MASA, *Transactions*, 1944, 29, MC 53, Folder 4.3, UAB.

4. Beardsley, *A History of Neglect*, 167.

5. Thomas, *Deluxe Jim Crow*, 89; Beardsley, *A History of Neglect*, 93, 94; See part 2 for more information on midwives' role in prenatal clinics, and part 3 for more on African American public health nurses.

6. Beardsley, *A History of Neglect*, 98, 99.

7. Beardsley, *A History of Neglect*, 170.

8. Dr. Helen Barnes, interview by Jenny Luke, Jackson, Mississippi, December 29, 2012.

9. Fraser, *African American Midwifery in the South*, 133.

10. Stabler, "The History of the Alabama Public Health System," 262.

11. MASA, *Transactions*, 1933, 10, RFHL.

12. MASA, *Transactions*, 1937, 12, RFHL.

13. MASA, *Transactions*, 1942, 12, RFHL.

14. Fraser, *African American Midwifery in the South*, 131.

15. Ward Jr., *Black Physicians in the Jim Crow South*, 170.

16. Thomas, *Deluxe Jim Crow*, 82.

17. Dr. Helen Barnes, interview by Jenny Luke, Jackson, Mississippi, December 29, 2012.

18. David Barton Smith, "The Politics of Racial Disparities," 257; Penfield Chester, *Sisters on a Journey: Portraits of American Midwives* (New Brunswick, NJ: Rutgers University Press, 1997), 139.

19. "Memphis Babies Born in Unsanitary Wards," *Chicago Defender (National Edition)*, August 19, 1944. ProQuest Historical Newspapers: Chicago Defender (1910–1975).

20. Sister Maria, R. S.M., "History of the Saint Martin de Porres Hospital, Mobile, Alabama," *Journal of the National Medical Association* 56, no. 4 (July 1964): 305.

21. Fraser, *African American Midwifery in the South*, 130–36.

22. Beardsley, *A History of Neglect*, 279.

23. Sandelowski, *Pain, Pleasure, and American Childbirth*, 61–70; Varney Burst and Thompson, *A History of Midwifery in the United States*, 95.

24. Joselyn Bacon, interview by Jenny Luke, Jackson, Mississippi, December 29, 2012.

25. Smith and Roberson, *My Bag Was Always Packed*, 117.

26. Chester, *Sisters on a Journey*, 139.

27. Smith and Roberson, *My Bag Was Always Packed*, 73. According to British obstetrician Grantly Dick Read, the reverse is true. The more women understand about the physiology of labor and what to expect, the less fear and therefore the less pain they experience. Considering childbirth a natural event may lessen the fear associated with it, but it obviously has no racial component.

28. Smith and Holmes, *Listen to Me Good*, 148.

29. Harriet A. Washington, *Medical Apartheid: The Dark History of Medical Experimentation on Black Americans from Colonial Times to the Present* (New York: First Anchor Books, 2006), 205.

30. Beardsley, *A History of Neglect*, 273–82.

31. MASA, *Transactions*, 1950, 5, RFHL.

32. Michael M. Davis and Hugh H. Smythe, "Providing Adequate Health Services to Negroes," *Journal of Negro Education* 18, no. 3, The Health Status and Health Education of Negroes in the United States (Summer 1949): 305–17.

33. For more on this program, see chapter 2.

34. Smith and Holmes, *Listen to Me Good*, 114. The infant mortality rate reflects the level of prenatal care.

CHAPTER 13. CHANGING CHILDBIRTH CUSTOMS

1. Fraser, *African American Midwifery in the South*, 166–67.

2. Smith and Holmes, *Listen to Me Good*, 155.

3. Smith and Roberson, *My Bag Was Always Packed*, 114.

4. Joselyn Bacon, interview, December 29, 2012.

5. Beardsley, *A History of Neglect*, 306.

6. Nelson, "Healthcare Reconsidered," 622; Beardsley, *A History of Neglect*, 307.

7. Karen L. Michaelson and Contributors, *Childbirth in America: Anthropological Perspectives* (South Hadley, Massachusetts: Bergin and Harvey, 1988), 55–65.

PART 4. MIDWIFERY IN TRANSITION

1. Debra Anne Susie, *The Way of Our Grandmothers: A Cultural View of Twentieth-Century Midwifery in Florida* (Athens: University of Georgia Press, 1988), 165.

2. Smith and Holmes, *Listen to Me Good*, 148.

3. Eugene R. Declercq, "The Transformation of American Midwifery: 1975 to 1988," *American Journal of Public Health* 82, no. 5 (1992): 681.

4. Mike Hollis, "Midwife Tradition Coming to an End in Rural Alabama," *Sunday-Star News*, 4C, January 6, 1985.

5. US Department of Health and Human Services, Health Resources and Services Administration, Maternal and Child Health Bureau, "Child Health USA 2014" (Rockville, MD: US Department of Health and Human Services, 2014). https://mchb.hrsa.gov/chusa14/health-services-financing-utilization/prenatal-care.html.

6. Geoffrey Warner, "Racial Differences in the Hurdling of Prenatal Care Barriers," *Review of Black Political Economy* 25, no. 3 (Winter 1997): 95–114.

7. Lesley Rathbun, telephone interview by Jenny Luke, July 6, 2015; Lesley Rathbun, e-mail update with author, August 7, 2017; www.charlestonbirthplace.com.

8. American College of Nurse-Midwives, *Annual Report 2104* (Silver Spring, MD: American College of Nurse-Midwives, 2014), 6.

CHAPTER 14. LAY MIDWIVES "RETIRE"

1. Bovard and Milton, *Why Not Me?* 38.

2. Beatrice Mongeau, Harvey L. Smith, and Ann C. Maney, "The 'Granny' Midwife: Changing Roles and Functions of a Folk Practitioner," *American Journal of Sociology* 66, no. 5 (March 1961): 505.

3. J. Clifton Edgar, "The Education, Licensing, and Supervision of the Midwife," *American Journal of Obstetrics and the Diseases of Women and Children* 73 (March 1916), in Judy Barrett Litoff, ed., *The American Midwife Debate: A Sourcebook on Its Modern Origins* (New York: Greenwood Press, 1986), 130.

4. E. R. Hardin, "The Midwife Problem," *Southern Medical Journal* 18 (May 1925), in Litoff, *The American Medical Debate*, 146.

5. Mongeau, Smith, and Maney, "The 'Granny' Midwife," 500.

6. L. S. B. Blachley, Letter to Florida State Board of Health, 1931, *Proposal to Discharge*, Series: S 900, Florida State Board of Health Subject Files, 1975–1975, Exhibits, Early Florida Medicine, State Library and Archives of Florida, https://www.floridamemory.com (accessed June 15, 2015).

7. South Carolina State Board of Health, *Lessons for Midwives*, South Carolina State Board of Health, revised 1970, 2, ARC.

8. Onnie Lee Logan quoted in Deborah Shelton Pinkney, "Onnie's Children: Mobile County's Last Lay Midwife, Onnie Lee Logan, Delivered Babies and Goodwill," *American Medical News* 33, no.15 (1990), www.cengage.com; see chapter 1, p. 27.

9. Smith and Holmes, *Listen to Me Good*, 101.

10. Smith and Holmes, *Listen to Me Good*, 145.

11. Smith and Holmes, *Listen to Me Good*, 100.

12. Alabama State Department of Public Health, *The Alabama Midwife: Her Book*, foreword.

13. Campbell, *Folks Do Get Born*, 90.

14. Campbell, *Folks Do Get Born*, 90.

15. Florida State Board of Health, *Discharge Certificate*, Exhibits, Early Florida Medicine, State Library and Archives of Florida, https://www.floridamemory.com (accessed June 15, 2015).

16. Campbell, *Folks Do Get Born*, 95.

17. Fraser, *African American Midwifery in the South*, 117; Campbell, *Folks Do Get Born*, 90.

18. Robert Loftus, "Stork Loses Two Long-Time Forrest County Helpers," *Hattiesburg (Miss.) American*, November 29, 1948, Midwife Program Files and Photographs—Public Health Nursing Division, 1911–1976, series 2036, box 8416, folder Midwife Supervision, MDAH.

19. Beardsley, *A History of Neglect*, 309.

20. Beardsley, *A History of Neglect*, 306. See chapter 11.

21. Institute of Medicine, Division of Health Promotion and Disease Prevention, Committee to Study Medical Professional Liability and the Delivery of Obstetric Care, *Medical Professional Liability and the Delivery of Obstetric Care, Volume 1* (Washington, DC: National Academy Press, 1989), 57–58.

22. Richard W. Wertz and Dorothy C. Wertz, *Lying-In: A History of Childbirth in America*, Expanded Edition (New Haven, CT: Yale University Press, 1989), 219.

23. Bovard and Milton, *Why Not Me?* 88–89.

24. Logan, *Motherwit*, 170.

25. Logan, *Motherwit*, 168.

26. Susie, *The Way of Our Grandmothers*, 137–59.

27. Holmes, "Louvenia Taylor Benjamin," 52.

28. Smith and Roberson, *My Bag Was Always Packed*, 126.

29. Logan, *Motherwit*, 173–74.

30. Ina Gaskin May, "Interview with Margaret Charles Smith," *Birth Gazette* 13, no. 1 (1996): 6.

31. Smith and Holmes, *Listen to Me Good*, 147.

32. Bovard and Milton, *Why Not Me?* 68–69; Milton Memorial Birthing Center, About Us, www.miltonmemorialbirthingcenter.com (accessed March 16, 2016).

33. Bovard and Milton, *Why Not Me?* 90.

34. Bovard and Milton, *Why Not Me?* 13–14.

35. Bovard and Milton, *Why Not Me?* 108–25; Katherine Griffin, "Gladys Delivers," *Health* 6, no. 3 (May 1992), http://www.eds.a.ebscohost.com.

36. Smith and Holmes, *Listen to Me Good*, 146.

37. Logan, *Motherwit*, 174.

38. Bovard and Milton, *Why Not Me?* 97.

CHAPTER 15. MIDWIFERY BECOMES A WHITE WOMAN'S REALM

1. Irene H. Butter and Bonnie J. Kay, "State Laws and the Practice of Midwifery," *American Journal of Public Health* 78, no. 9 (1988): 1161.

2. Declercq, "The Transformation of American Midwifery: 1975 to 1988," 680.

3. Goan, *Mary Breckinridge*, 235–36; Ettinger, *Nurse-Midwifery*, 180–85; Varney and Thompson, *A History of Midwifery in the United States*, 162.

4. Goan, *Mary Breckinridge*, 101.

5. Ettinger, *Nurse-Midwifery*, 180; Varney and Thompson, *A History of Midwifery in the United States*, 162.

6. Goan, *Mary Breckinridge*, 236; Ettinger, *Nurse-Midwifery*, 183; Varney and Thompson, *A History of Midwifery in the United States*, 161.

7. Katherine Louise Dawley, "Leaving the Nest: Nurse-Midwifery in the United States, 1940–1980" (PhD diss., University of Pennsylvania, 2001), 79.

8. Ettinger, *Nurse-Midwifery*, 187.

9. Joselyn Bacon, in an interview by Jenny Luke, Jackson, Mississippi, December 29, 2012.

10. Margaret Morton and Edna R. Roberts, "Celebrating Public Health Nursing: Caring for Mississippi's Communities with Courage and Compassion, 1920–1993," *Mississippi Department of Health*, http://msdh.ms.gov/msdhsite/_static/19,10778,378.html#; J. Edward Hill, *The State of American Medicine*, speech as immediate past president to the American Medical Association, The Denver Forum, October 25, 2006, http://www.thedenverforum.com/recent-speeches/the-state-of-american-medicine/.

11. Dr. J. Edward Hill, interview by Jenny Luke, Tupelo, Mississippi, May 15, 2017.

12. Dr. Helen Barnes, interview by Jenny Luke, Jackson, Mississippi, December 29, 2012; Dr. J. Edward Hill, interview by Jenny Luke, Tupelo, Mississippi, May 15, 2017.

13. Varney and Thompson, *A History of Midwifery in the United States*, 128.

14. Ettinger, *Nurse-Midwifery*, 189; Varney and Thompson, *A History of Midwifery in the United States*, 192.

15. US Government House of Representatives, Nurse-Midwifery: Consumers' Freedom of Choice hearing before the subcommittee on oversight and investigations of the Committee on Interstate and Foreign Commerce, Dec. 18, 1980 (Washington, DC: US Government Printing Office, 1981), the testimony of Sally Tom, CNM, MC 53, 4.91, UAB.

16. Cynthia Rector Air, interviewed by Anita Smith, October 24, 1996, School of Nursing Oral History Collection, UAB. Cynthia Air was the president of the Alabama Nurses Association, 1978–1980.

17. Mary Ann Shah, "The Unification of Midwives: A Time for Dialogue," *Journal of Nurse-Midwifery* 27, no. 5 (September/October 1982): 1–2.

18. ACNM, State Fact Sheets, http://www.midwife.org/State-Fact-Sheets (accessed August 23, 2017). Figures are for 2013.

19. Y. Tony Yang, Laura B. Attanasio, and Katy B. Kozhimannil, "State Scope of Practice Laws, Nurse-Midwifery Workforce, and Childbirth Procedures and Outcome," *Women's Health Issues* 26, no. 3 (2016): 266. https://doi.org/10.1016/j.whi2016.02.003 (accessed August 23, 2017).

20. ACNM, State Fact Sheets; Eugene Declercq, "Birth Attended by Certified Nurse-Midwives in the United States in 2005," *Journal of Midwifery and Women's Health* 54, no. 1 (January/February 2009): 95; Ettinger, *Nurse-Midwifery*, 193. In 2014, there were 11,475 CNMs and 103 CMs; they attended 91.3 percent of all midwife-attended births, 8.3 percent of total US births.

21. America's Health Ranking, "Infant mortality by state, 2015," United Health Foundation, 2017, https://www.americashealthrankings.org/explore/2015-annual-report/measure/IMR/state/ALL (accessed August 23, 2017).

CHAPTER 16. MIDWIFERY TODAY AND ITS POTENTIAL FOR TOMORROW

1. American College of Nurse Midwives (ACNM), *Fact Sheet: Essential Facts about Midwives*, http://www.midwife.org/acnm/files/ccLibraryFiles/Filename/000000005463/EssentialFactsAboutMidwivesJune2015.pdf (accessed July 24, 2015); ACNM, *Annual Report, 2014* (Silver Spring, MD: ACNM, 2014), 9.

2. Dr. Heather Clarke, telephone interview by Jenny Luke, March 21, 2016.

3. ACNM, *Annual Report, 2014*, 9.

4. ACNM, *Fact Sheet*; ACNM, *Midwifery: Evidence Based Practice—A Summary of Research on Midwifery Practice in the United States* (Silver Spring, MD: ACNM, 2012), www.midwife.org; Helen Varney Burst, "History of Nurse-Midwifery in Reproductive Healthcare," *Journal of Nurse-Midwifery* 43, no. 6 (November/December 1998), par. 14, 22, http://www.sciencedirect.com.

5. T. J. Mathews and M. F. MacDorman, "Infant Mortality Statistics from the 2010 Period Linked Birth/Infant Death Data Set," *National Vital Statistics Reports* 62, no. 8 (Hyattsville, MD: National Center for Health Statistics, 2013). http://www.cdc.gov/nchs/data/nvsr/nvsr62/nvsr62_08.pdf.

6. Marjorie Morgan, "Prenatal Care of African American Women in Selected USA Urban and Rural Cultural Contexts," *Journal of Transcultural Nursing* 7, no. 2 (January–June 1996): 5–7.

7. Geoffrey Warner, "Racial Differences in the Hurdling of Prenatal Care Barriers," *Review of Black Political Economy* 25, no. 3 (Winter 1997): 109–10.

8. Dr. Heather Clarke, telephone interview by Jenny Luke, March 21, 2016.

9. Linda Janet Holmes, *Into the Light of Day: Reflections on the History of Midwives of Color within the American College of Nurse-Midwives* (Silver Spring, MD: American College of Nurse-Midwives, 2012), 16.

10. Holmes, *Into the Light of Day*.

11. Holmes, *Into the Light of Day*, 25.

12. Holmes, *Into the Light of Day*, 30.

13. Holmes, *Into the Light of Day*, 26.

14. Anitra Ellerby-Brown, Trickera Sims, and Mavis Schorn, "African American Nurse-Midwives: Continuing the Legacy," *Minority Nurse* (Fall 2008), https://www.nursing.vanderbilt.edu/msn/pdf/nmw_midwiferyforAA.pdf (accessed June 15, 2015); Dr. Heather Clarke, telephone interview by Jenny Luke, March 21, 2016; ACNM, *Forging Our Future: An Invitation to Preview the Proposed ACNM 2015–2020 Strategic Plan*, http://www.midwife.org/acnm/files/ccLibraryFiles/Filename/000000005133/ACNM-Executive-Summary-of-Draft-Strat-Plan-Apr2015.pdf (accessed June 16, 2015).

15. Varney and Thompson, *A History of Midwifery in the United States*, 154.

16. Approximate tuition taken from the Frontier Nursing University website, www.frontier.edu.

17. Holmes, *Into the Light of Day*, 19.

18. International Center for Traditional Childbearing, *About ICTC*, www.ictcmidwvies .org; Dr. Heather Clarke, interview by Jenny Luke, March 21, 2016.

19. Dr. J. Edward Hill, interview by Jenny Luke, May 15, 2017.

20. International Center for Traditional Childbearing, *About ICTC*, www.ictcmidwvies .org; Dr. Heather Clarke, interview by Jenny Luke, March 21, 2016; Jamarah Amani, "Continuing the Tradition: Becoming a Midwife with Jamarah Amani," *State of Black Midwifery Summit* (MP3), December 7, 2013, www.senadamarketing.com.

21. Jamarah Amani, "Continuing the Tradition: Becoming a Midwife with Jamarah Amani," *State of Black Midwifery Summit* (MP3), December 7, 2013, www.senadamarket ing.com; Circle of Mamas program, www.southernbirthjustice.org (accessed March 24, 2016); Maria Milton, "Milton Memorial Birth Center: Continuing the Legacy of Black Midwifery in Florida," *State of Black Midwifery Summit* (MP3), December 7, 2013, www .senadamarketing.com.

22. JayVon Muhammed, "Public Health Policies and Doing for Self," *State of Black Midwifery Summit* (MP3), December 7, 2013, www.senadamarketing.com.

23. Dr. Heather Clarke, interview by Jenny Luke, March 21, 2016.

24. Kimberley Allers Seals, "Midwifery's Diversity Problem Hits Spotlight," *Women's eNews*, August 14, 2015, http://womensenews.org/2015/08/midwiferys-diversity-problem -hits-spotlight/, US MERA, *US MERA Statement of Commitment to Health Equity in Maternal and Newborn Health and to Greater Diversity in Midwifery*, September 15, 2015, www.usmera.org (accessed March 25, 2016).

25. US MERA, *US MERA Welcomes International Center for Traditional Childbearing (ICTC) to the Coalition*, February 11, 2016, www.usmera.org (accessed March 25, 2016).

EPILOGUE

1. Rhonda Pines, "Margaret Charles Smith: She Knows Motherhood by Heart," *Tuscaloosa News*, May 12, 1985, http://news.google.com/newspapers?nid=1817&dat= 19850512&id=dSkoAAAAIBAJ&sjid=1KUEAAAAIBAJ&pg=1446,4215918 (accessed January 22, 2016); Paul, *Miss Margaret*, DVD; The International Center for Traditional Childbearing, *About ICTC*, http://ictcmidwives.org/about-ictc/ictc-history/ (accessed January 22, 2016).

2. Logan, *Motherwit*, ix.

3. ACNM, *Fact Sheet*.

4. Helen Varney Burst, "Two Roads—Which One?" *Journal of Nurse-Midwifery* 26, no. 5 (September/October 1981): 7–12.

5. American College of Nurse-Midwives, *Midwifery: Evidence Based Practice, 2012* (Silver Spring, MD: American College of Nurse-Midwives, 2012). www.midwife.org.

6. ACNM, *Forging Our Future: ACNM 2015–2020 Strategic Plan* (Silver Spring, 2015), 3 http://www.midwife.org/ACNM/files/ccLibraryFiles/FILENAME/000000005401/2015-20-strategicplanexecsummary-final-070915.pdf (accessed July 24, 2015).

7. US MERA, *2015 Annual Meeting Report*, http://www.midwife.org/acnm/files/ccLibraryFiles/FILENAME/000000005443/US-MERA-2015-Annual-Meeting-Report-Final.pdf.

8. Jamie Santa Cruz, "Call the Midwife," *Atlantic*, June 12, 2015, http://www.theatlantic.com/health/archive/2015/06/midwives-are-making-a-comeback/395456/ (accessed July 24, 2015).

9. Cruz, "Call the Midwife."

10. Cruz, "Call the Midwife."

11. J. Edward Hill, *The State of American Medicine*, speech; Dr. J. Edward Hill, interview by Jenny Luke, May 15, 2017.

12. Thomas M. Boulware, interviewed by Virginia Fisher, June 30, 1987, MC 45, Folder 1.17, UAB.

13. "Advancing Medicine," *Southwestern Medicine Annual Review, 2015*, 25, no. 1 (March 2016): 40. Barber Assisted Reduction in Blood Pressure in Ethnic Residents (BARBER-1). When M. O. Bousfield MD addressed the annual meeting of the American Public Health Association in 1933, he listed the barber as one of the access points for disseminating health education to the African American community.

14. J. Edward Hill, *The State of American Medicine*, speech.

BIBLIOGRAPHY

ARCHIVAL COLLECTIONS AND DOCUMENTS

Alabama Department of Archives and History (ADAH)

(All in Datcher Family Collection, LPR 315. Box 2. Folder 8)
"Demonstration of Preparation for Delivery." Packet of Instructions. Montgomery, Alabama: Alabama State Department of Health, Bureau of Maternal and Child Health, 1950s.
"A General Daily Guide during Normal Pregnancy." Packet of Instructions. Bureau of Maternal and Child Health, 1958.
"Oral Quiz for Midwives." Montgomery, Alabama: Alabama State Department of Health, Bureau of Maternal and Child Health, 1950s.
"Prenatal Instructions for Cases Attended by Midwives." Packet of Instructions. Bureau of Maternal and Child Health, 1955.

Elizabeth M Bear Collection, Avery Research Center (ARC)

Bulletin of the Tuskegee School of Nurse-Midwifery. Tuskegee Institute, Alabama, 1945.
Lessons for Midwives. South Carolina State Board of Health, revised 1970.
Papers from Series 1: Nurse-Midwives, 1941–2006.
Papers from Series 2: Penn Center.
"Standing Orders." Macon County Health Department, revised 1945.

Mississippi Department of Archives and History (MDAH)

(Series 2036/Box 8416)
Collection: Midwife Program Files and Photographs—Public Health Nursing Division, 1911–1976.
"Leflore Midwife Fails on Fee, Takes Baby." *Jackson Daily News.* November 8, 1939.
Lesson Outlines for Teaching Midwives. Jackson, MS: State Board of Public Health, 1939(?).

Manual for Midwives. State Board of Health. Jackson, MS: Mississippi State Board of Health, 19— (1931[?]).

Mississippi State Board of Health. "Teaching Guide—Midwife Supervision." Division of Public Health Nursing, Mississippi State Board of Health, Jackson, Mississippi, 1962.

Mississippi State Board of Health. "Relation of the Midwife to the State Board of Health." Mississippi State Board of Health, 1931.

Mississippi State Board of Health. "Relation of the Midwife to the State Board of Health." Mississippi State Board of Health, 1938(?).

University of Alabama Reynolds-Finley Historical Library (RFHL)

Gewin, W. C. "Careless and unscientific midwifery with Special References to some features of the work of Midwives." *The Alabama Medical Journal.* Series 4, Vol. 11 (1905–1906): 629–35.

Jones, Anita M. *Manual for Teaching Midwives.* Washington, DC: United States Department of Labor, Children's Bureau, 1941.

Transactions of the Medical Association of the State of Alabama. "Reports from the Committee on Maternal and Child Health." Montgomery: Medical Association of the State of Alabama, 1933–1956.

Wilkinson, D. L. "Alabama's need of more Stringent Midwifery laws." *Transactions of the Medical Association of Alabama,* 1898.

University of Alabama at Birmingham Archives (UAB)

Air, Cynthia Rector. Interviewed by Anita Smith, October 24, 1996. School of Nursing Oral History Collection.

Boulware Draft (written as a history of Boulware in Birmingham), MC53 Box 4 Folder 15 Tom Boulware Collection, MC33 Box 1 Folder 1.

Boulware, T. M., Elizabeth LaForge, and R. C. Stewart. "A Negro Demonstration Center for Maternal and Newborn Care in Alabama." *Southern Medical Association* 36, no. 12 (December 1943): 784–91.

Harrison, Tinsley R., MD. Letter to Brewer Dixon. May 7, 1951. MC 53 4.35.

Maternal Mortality in Birmingham, and Jefferson County, Alabama, 1931–1935. Joint Report of the Jefferson Co. Medical Society & Jefferson Co. Board of Health, 1936.

Montgomery, James T., MD. Interviewed by Virginia Fisher, August 26, 1987. MC45 1.45.

A Report on the Five-year Study of Maternal Mortality in Alabama, 1944–1948. Committee on Maternal and Child Health of the Medical Association of the State of Alabama.

Transactions of the Medical Association of the State of Alabama. (Reports on Tuskegee School of Nurse-Midwifery, Slossfield Hospital, Cullman County Maternity Program.) Montgomery: Medical Association of the State of Alabama, 1943–1949.

Underwood, Felix J. "The Development of Midwifery in Mississippi." *Southern Medical Journal* (September 1926): 683–84.

US Government House of Representatives. *Nurse-Midwifery: Consumers' Freedom of Choice hearing before the subcommittee on oversight and investigations of the Committee on Interstate and Foreign Commerce*, Dec. 18, 1980. Washington, DC: GPO, 1981. MC 53 Box 4 Folder 91.

PRIMARY SOURCES

Alabama Department of Public Health. Live Births with Adequate and Less than Adequate Prenatal Care, According to the Adequacy of Prenatal Care Utilization (Kotelchuck) Index, by Race of Mother, County and Perinatal Region of Residence Alabama, 2012. http://adph.org/healthstats/assets/mch12_9.pdf.

———. Alabama Department of Public Health 1969 Activities Report. Montgomery: Alabama Department of Public Health, 1969.

———. Alabama Department of Public Health 2011 Annual Report. Montgomery, AL: Bureau of Health Promotion and Chronic Disease, 2011. http://www.adph.org/publications/assets/2011annrpt.pdf.

———. Alabama Department of Public Health 2013 Annual Report. Montgomery, AL: Bureau of Health Promotion and Chronic Disease, 2013. http://www.adph.org/publications/assets/2013annrpt.pdf.

———. *The Alabama Midwife: Her Book*. Montgomery: Alabama State Department of Public Health, 1956.

All My Babies: A Midwife's Own Story. Film. Directed by George C. Stoney. Atlanta: Georgia Department of Public Health, 1953.

Amani, Jamarah. "Continuing the Tradition: Becoming a Midwife with Jamarah Amani." *State of Black Midwifery Summit*. (MP3). December 7, 2013. www.senadamarketing.com.

American College of Nurse-Midwives. *Midwifery: Evidence Based Practice, A Summary of Research on Midwifery Practice in the United States, 2012*. Silver Spring, MD. www.midwife.org.

———. *Fact Sheet: Essential Facts about Midwives, 2015*. Silver Spring, MD. www.midwife.org.

———. *Annual Report 2014: Global Spotlight on Midwives: Driving Change at Home and Around the World*. Silver Spring, MD. http://www.midwife.org/ACNM-Annual-Reports.

———. *State Fact Sheets*, http://www.midwife.org/State-Fact-Sheets.

———. *Improving Access to Maternity Care Act 2015 (H.R. 1209/S.628)*. Silver Spring, MD, 2015. http://www.midwife.org/acnm/files/ccLibraryFiles/Filename/000000005035/MaternityShortageAreaLegislationTPs.pdf.

———. *Forging Our Future: An Invitation to Preview the Proposed ACNM 2015–2020 Strategic Plan*, http://www.midwife.org/acnm/files/ccLibraryFiles/Filename/000000005133/ACNM-Executive-Summary-of-Draft-Strat-Plan-Apr2015.pdf.

American Congress of Obstetrics and Gynecology (ACOG). *ACOG Endorses the International Confederation of Midwives Standards for Midwifery Education, Training, Licensure, and Regulation*. April 20, 2015. Washington, DC. www.acog.org.

———. *ACOG Applauds Introduction to Improving Access to Maternity Care Act*. March 3, 2015. Washington, DC. www.acog.org.

———. *"AIM"ing to Reduce U.S. Maternal Mortality*. Posted October 24, 2016.

America's Health Ranking. "Infant mortality by state, 2015." United Health Foundation, 2017. https://www.americashealthrankings.org/explore/2015-annual-report/measure/IMR/state/ALL.

———. "Florida Battles High Death Rates in Maternity Cases." *Chicago Defender (National Edition)*, December 28, 1946.

———. "Memphis Babies Born in Unsanitary Wards." *Chicago Defender (National Edition)*, August 19, 1944.

———. "Says Women Sent Home Two Hours after Having Babies at Freedman's." *Chicago Defender (National Edition)*, March 1, 1952.

Abbott, Grace. "Federal Aid for the Protection of Maternity and Infancy." *American Journal of Public Health* 12, no. 9 (September 1922): 737–42. http://ajph.aphapublications.org/doi/pdf/10.2105/AJPH.12.9.737-a.

Bacon, Joselyn. Interview by Jenny Luke. Jackson, Mississippi, December 29, 2012.

Barnes, Helen. Interview by Jenny Luke. Jackson, Mississippi, December 29, 2012.

Blachley, L. S. B. Letter to Florida State Board of Health, 1931. *Proposal to Discharge*. Series: S 900- Florida State Board of Health Subject files, 1875–1975. Florida Memory: State Library and Archives of Florida. www.floridamemory.com/exhibits/medicine/midwives.

Blackburn, Laura. "The Midwife as an Ally." *American Journal of Nursing* 42, no. 1 (1942): 57. www.jstor.org.

———. "The Midwife Problem in Rural Areas of the South." *Trained Nurse and Hospital Review* (1939): 128–30.

Bousfield, M. O. "Reaching the Negro Community." *American Journal of Public Health* 24, no. 3 (March 1934): 209–15. http://ajph.aphapublications.org/doi/pdf/10.2105/AJPH.24.3.209.

Bovard, Wendy, and Gladys Milton. *Why Not Me? The Story of Gladys Milton, Midwife*. Summertown, TN: The Book Publishing Company, 1993.

Breckinridge, Mary. *Wide Neighborhoods: A Story of the Frontier Nursing Service*. Lexington: University of Kentucky Press, 1981.

The Center for Traditional Childbearing. *About Us*. http://ictcmidwives.org/history/.

Chambers, Jesse. "Screening of 'Miss Margaret' Documentary in Eutaw." *Birmingham Weekly.* http://bhamweekly.com/birmingham/article-737-screening-of-miss-mar garet-documentary-in-eutaw.html (accessed June 15, 2012).

Clarke, Heather. Telephone interview by Jenny Luke. March 21, 2106.

Conner, Douglas L., with John F. Marszalek. *A Black Physician's Story: Bringing Hope in Mississippi.* Jackson: University Press of Mississippi, 1985.

Davis, Michael M., and Hugh H. Smythe. "Providing Adequate Health Service to Negroes." *Journal of Negro Education* 18, no. 3 (1949): 305–17.

Dribble, Eugene H., Jr., MD, Louis A. Rabb, and Ruth B. Ballard. "John A. Andrew Memorial Hospital." *Journal of the National Medical Association* 53, no. 2 (March 1961): 103–18.

Ferguson, James H. "Mississippi Midwives." *Journal of the History of Medicine* (Winter 1950): 85–95.

Florida State Board of Health. *Discharge Certificate.* Series: S 900—Florida State Board of Health Subject files, 1875–1975. Florida Memory: State Library and Archives of Florida. www.floridamemory.com/exhibits/medicine/midwives.

Gaskin, Ina May. "Interview with Margaret Charles Smith." *Birth Gazette* 13, no.1 (Winter 1996). http://eds.b.ebscohost.com.

Hill, J. Edward. "The State of American Medicine." *The Denver Forum.* Speech to American Medical Association, October 25, 2006. http://www.thedenverforum .com/recent-speeches/the-state-of-american-medicine/.

Hill, J. Edward. Personal interview by Jenny Luke. Tupelo, Mississippi. May 15, 2017.

Hilliard, Mary B. Interviewed by Daisy M. Greene. October 19, 1977. Oral History Project. Mississippi Department of Archives and History. Jackson, Mississippi.

Holmes, Linda Janet. "Louvenia Taylor Benjamin, Southern Lay Midwife: An Interview." *Sage* 2, no. 2 (Fall 1985): 51–54.

Jacobsen, Paul H. "Hospital Care and the Vanishing Midwife." *Millbank Memorial Fund Quarterly* 34, no. 3 (1956): 253–61.

Kenney, John A. "The First Graduating Class of the Tuskegee School of Midwifery." *Journal of the National Medical Association* 34, no. 3 (1942): 107–9.

Kerr, Jill Shatzen. "Burgess Leads Bipartisan Group in Introducing Bill to Improve Access to Maternity Care." *Blog.* March 3, 2015. US Congressman Michael C. Burgess, MD. Serving the 26th District of Texas. www.burgess.house.gov/blog.

Litoff, Judy Barrett. *The American Midwife Debate: A Sourcebook on Its Modern Origins.* Contributions in Medical Studies, Number 18. New York: Greenwood Press, 1986.

Logan, Onnie Lee, and Katherine Clark. *Motherwit: An Alabama Midwife's Story.* New York: E. P. Dutton, 1989.

Maddux, Walter H. "The Slossfield Health Center: An Example of Local Medical Service for Mothers and Children under Public Health Auspices." *American Journal of Public Health* 31 (May1941): 481–86.

Maron, Diana Fine. "Has Maternal Mortality Really Doubled in the U.S.?" *Scientific American*, June 8, 2015. http://www.scientificamerican.com/article/has-maternal -mortality-really-doubled-in-the-u-s/.

Maternity Center Association. *Twenty Years of Nurse-Midwifery, 1933–1953*. New York: Maternity Center Association, 1955.

Mathews, T. J., and M. F. MacDorman. "Infant Mortality Statistics from the 2010 period linked birth/infant death data set." *National Vital Statistics Reports* 62, no. 8. Hyattsville, MD: National Center for Health Statistics, 2013. http://www.cdc.gov/ nchs/data/nvsr/nvsr62/nvsr62_08.pdf.

Milton Memorial Birthing Center. www.miltonmemorialbirthingcenter.com.

Milton, Maria. "Milton Memorial Birth Center: Continuing the Legacy of Black Midwifery in Florida." *State of Black Midwifery Summit*. (MP3). December 7, 2013. www.senadamarketing.com.

Muhammed, JayVon. "Public Health Policies and Doing for Self." *State of Black Midwifery Summit*. (MP3). December 7, 2013. www.senadamarketing.com.

Pines, Rhonda. "Margaret Charles Smith: She Knows Motherhood by Heart." *Tuscaloosa News*. May 12, 1985. http://news.google.com/newspapers?nid=1817&dat=19850512&i d=dSkoAAAAIBAJ&sjid=1KUEAAAAIBAJ&pg=1446,4215918.

Pinkney, Deborah Shelton. "Onnie's Children; Mobile County's Last Lay Midwife, Onnie Lee Logan, Delivered Babies and Goodwill." *American Medical News* 33, no. 15 (April 20, 1990). http://galenet.galegroup.com.

Rathbun, Lesley. Phone interview by Jenny Luke. July 6, 2015.

Riddle, Estelle G. Massey. "The Progress of Negro Nursing." *American Journal of Nursing* 38, no. 2 (1938): 162–69.

———. "The Training and Placement of Negro Nurses." *Journal of Negro Education* 4, no. 1 (1935): 42–48.

Rothert, Frances Catherine. *Maternal Mortality in Fifteen States*. Washington, DC: Department of Labor, Children's Bureau, 1934.

Santa Cruz, Jamie. "Call the Midwife." *Atlantic*. June 12, 2015. www.theatlantic.com/ health/archive/2015/06/midwives-are-making-a-comeback/395456.

Seals, Kimberley Allers. "Midwifery's Diversity Problem Hits Spotlight." *Women's eNews*, August 14, 2015. http://womensenews.org/2015/08/midwiferys-diversity -hits-spotlight/.

Sebastian, S. P. "The L. Richardson Memorial Hospital." *Journal of the National Medical Association* 22, no. 3 (1930): 142–44.

Sister Maria, R. S.M. "History of the Saint Martin De Porres Hospital, Mobile, Alabama." *Journal of the National Medical Association* 56, no. 4 (1964): 302–6.

Smith, Claudine Curry, and Mildred H. Roberson. *My Bag Was Always Packed: The Life and Times of a Virginia Midwife*. Bloomington, IN: 1st Books, 2003.

Smith, Margaret Charles, and Linda Janet Holmes. *Listen to Me Good: The Life Story of an Alabama Midwife*. Women and Health Series. Edited by Rima D. Apple and Janet Golden. Columbus: Ohio State University Press, 1996.

Smith, W. Eugene. "Nurse-Midwife: Maude Callen Eases the Pain of Birth, Life, and Death." *Life*. December 3, 1951. 134–45.

Southern Rural Black Women's Initiative. "Unequal Lives: The State of Black Women and Families in the Rural South." http://srbwi.org/index.php?/news.

Southwestern Medicine. *Advancing Medicine* 25, no. 1 (March 2016). University of Texas Southwestern Medical Center. Dallas, Texas.

Stabler, Carey V. "The History of the Alabama Public Health System." PhD diss., Duke University, 1944.

Stoney, George C. *All My Babies: A Midwife's Own Story*. Film directed by George C. Stoney. Atlanta: Georgia Department of Public Health, 1953.

The Story of an Alabama Granny Midwife. DVD. Directed by Diana Paul. 2010; Tiburon, CA: Sage Femme.

Thomas, Margaret W. "School for Negro Nurse-Midwives." *American Journal of Nursing* 44, no. 9 (1944): 914.

Thomas, Robert McG., Jr. "Onnie Lee Logan, 85, Midwife Whose 'Motherwit' Drew Praise." *New York Times*. July 13, 1995. Obituaries. http://nytimes.com/1995/07/13/obituaries/onnie-lee-logan-85-midwife-whose-motherwit-drew-praise.html.

Tuskegee Institute, Alabama. "Bulletin of the Tuskegee School of Nurse-Midwifery, 1945." *Smith Libraries Exhibits*. https://libex.smith.edu/omeka/items/show/478 (accessed April 22, 2016).

US Commission on Civil Rights. *Title VI . . . One Year After: A Survey of Desegregation of Health and Welfare Services in the South, 1966*. Washington, DC: US Government Printing Office, 1966.

US Department of Health and Human Services. Health Resources and Services Administration. Maternal and Child Health Bureau. *Child Health USA 2013*. Rockville, MD: US Department of Health and Human Services, 2013.

US Department of Health and Human Services. Health Resources and Services Administration. Maternal and Child Health Bureau. *Child Health USA 2014*. Rockville, MD: US Department of Health and Human Services, 2014. https://mchb.hrsa.gov/chusa14/health-services-financing-utilization/prenatalcare.html.

US Midwifery Education, Regulation, and Association. *US MERA Statement of Commitment to Health Equity in Maternal and Newborn Health and to Greater Diversity in Midwifery*. September 15, 2015. www.usmera.org (accessed March 25, 2016).

US Midwifery Education, Regulation, and Association. *US MERA Welcomes International Center for Traditional Childbearing (ICTC) to the Coalition*. February 11, 2016. www.usmera.org (accessed March 25, 2016).

Varney Burst, Helen. "Two Roads—Which One?" *Journal of Nurse-Midwifery* 26, no. 5 (September/October 1981): 7–12.

Wallace, Kelly. "Why Is the Maternal Mortality Rate Going Up in the United States?" *Cable News Network* (CNN). December 11, 2015. http://www.cnn.com/2015/12/01/health/maternal-mortality-rate-u-s-increasing-why/.

Walton, Marsha. "Doctors Open Window on U.S. Maternal Care Crisis." *Women's eNews*, November 1, 2015. http://womensenews.org/2015/11/doctors-open-window-on-u-s-maternal-care-crisis/.

SECONDARY SOURCES

Airhihenbuwa, Collins O., and Leandris Liburd. "Eliminating Health Disparities: The Interface of Culture, Gender, and Power." *Health Education and Behavior* 33, no. 4 (2006): 488–501.

Amnesty International. *Deadly Delivery: The Maternal Health Care Crisis in the USA.* London, UK: Amnesty International Secretariat, 2010.

Barney, Sandra Lee. *Authorized to Heal: Gender, Class, and the Transformation of Medicine in Appalachia, 1880–1930.* Chapel Hill: University of North Carolina Press, 2000.

Barry, Detrice G., and Joyceen S. Boyle. "An Ethnohistory of a Granny Midwife." *Journal of Transcultural Nursing* 8, no. 1 (December 1996): 13–18.

Beardsley, Edward H. *A History of Neglect: Healthcare for Blacks and Mill Workers in the Twentieth-Century South.* Knoxville: University of Tennessee Press, 1987.

———. "Desegregating Southern Medicine, 1945–1970." *International Social Science Review* 71, no. 1/2 (1996): 37–54. www.jstor.org.

Beito, David T., and Linda Royster Beito. "Let Down Your Bucket Where You Are: The Afro-American Hospital and Black Health Care in Mississippi, 1924–1966." *Social Science History* 30, no. 4 (2006): 551–69.

Bell, Pegge L. "'Making Do' with the Midwife: Arkansas' Mamie O. Hale in the 1940s." *Nursing History Review: Official Journal of the American Association for the History of Nursing* 1 (1993): 155–69.

———. "Mamie Odessa Hale Garland (1911–1968?)." The Central Arkansas Library System, http://encyclopediaofarkansas.net/encyclopedia/entry-detail.aspx?entryID=1662 (accessed August 15, 2012).

Blair, Barbara, and Susan E. Cayleff, ed. *Wings of Gauze: Women of Color and the Experience of Health and Illness.* Detroit: Wayne State University Press, 1993.

Bridgforth, Lucie Robertson. "The Politics of Public Health Reform: Felix J. Underwood and the Mississippi State Board of Health, 1924–58." *Public Historian* 6, no. 3 (Summer 1984): 5–26.

Butter, Irene H., and Bonnie J. Kay. "State Laws and the Practice of Lay Midwifery." *American Journal of Public Health* 78, no. 9 (September 1988): 1161–69.

Campbell, Marie. *Folks Do Get Born*. New York: Rinehart and Company, 1946.

Canty, Lucinda. "The Graduates of the Tuskegee School of Nurse-Midwifery." Master's thesis, Yale University, 1994.

Carnegie, Mary Elizabeth. *The Path We Tread: Blacks in Nursing, 1854–1984*. Philadelphia, PA: J. B. Lippincott, 1986.

Cavender, Anthony. "A Midwife's Commonplace Book." *Appalachia Journal* 32, no. 2 (Winter 2005): 182–90.

Chester, Penfield. *Sisters on a Journey: Portraits of American Midwives*. New Brunswick, NJ: Rutgers University Press, 1995.

Clarke, Ann L. *Culture Childbearing Health Professionals*. Philadelphia: F. A. Davis Company, 1978.

Cobb, James C. *The Most Southern Place on Earth: The Mississippi Delta and the Roots of Regional Identity*. Oxford: Oxford University Press, 1992.

Conlon, Sarah. "A Hospital Built by Them, for Them: The Good Samaritan Waverly Hospital Building Fund Campaign and the Evolution of Black Health Care Traditions in South Carolina." Thesis, University of South Carolina, 2012.

Davis, Althea T. *Early Black Leaders in Nursing: Architects for Integration and Equality*. National League for Nursing Series. Sudbury, MA: Jones and Bartlett, 1999.

Dawley, Katherine Louise. "Leaving the Nest: Nurse-Midwifery in the United States, 1940–1980." PhD diss., University of Pennsylvania, 2001.

Declercq, Eugene R. "The Transformation of American Midwifery: 1975 to 1988." *American Journal of Public Health* 82 (1992): 680–84.

——. "Births Attended by Certified Nurse-Midwives in the United States in 2005." *Journal of Midwifery and Women's Health* 54, no. 1 (January/February 2009): 95–96.

Downs, Jim. *Sick from Freedom: African-American Illness and Suffering during the Civil War and Reconstruction*. New York: Oxford University Press, 2012.

Eakins, Pamela S., ed. *The American Way of Birth*. Philadelphia: Temple University Press, 1986.

Ellerby-Brown, Anitra, and Trickera Sims. "African American Nurse-Midwives: Continuing the Legacy." *Minority Nurse* (Fall 2008): 46–49.

Ettinger, Laura E. *Nurse-Midwifery: The Birth of a New American Profession*. Women, Gender, and Health. Edited by Susan L. Smith and Nancy Tomes. Columbus: Ohio State University Press, 2006.

Fett, Sharla M. *Working Cures: Health, Healing, and Power on Southern Slave Plantations*. Chapel Hill: University of North Carolina Press, 2002.

Fraser, Gertrude Jacinta. *African American Midwifery in the South: Dialogues of Birth, Race, and Memory*. Cambridge, MA: Harvard University Press, 1998.

Gamble, Vanessa Northington. *Making a Place for Ourselves: The Black Hospital Movement, 1920–1950*. New York: Oxford University Press, 1995.

Goan, Melanie Beals. *Mary Breckinridge: The Frontier Nursing Service and Rural Health in Appalachia.* Chapel Hill: University of North Carolina Press, 2008.

Graninger, Elizabeth. "Granny-Midwives: Matriarchs of Birth in the African American Community 1600–1940." *Birth Gazette* 13, no. 1 (Winter 1996): 9, http://eds.b.ebscohost .com

Griffin, Katherine. "Gladys Delivers." *Health* 6, no. 3 (May 1992). http://eds.a.ebscohost .com.

Harakas, Margo. "Women Making a Difference." *Orlando Sentinel,* June 7, 1998. http:// articles.orlandosentinel.com.

Hill, Patricia Evridge. "Dr. Hilla Sheriff: Caught between Science and the State at the South Carolina Midwife Training Institutes." In *South Carolina Women: Their Lives and Times, Volume 3.* Edited by Marjorie Julian Spruill, Valinda W. Littlefield, and Joan Marie Johnson. Athens: University of Georgia Press, 2012.

———. "Review of Fraser, Gertrude Jacinta." *African American Midwifery in the South: Dialogues of Birth, Race and Memory.* H-Net: Humanities & Social Sciences Online, http://www.h-net.org/reviews/showrev.php?id=3642 (accessed August 25, 2012).

Hine, Darlene Clark. "African American Women and Their Communities in the Twentieth Century." *Black Women, Gender + Families* 1, no. 1 (2007): 1–23.

———. *Black Women in the Nursing Profession: A Documentary History.* The History of American Nursing. Edited by Susan Reverby. 16th edition. New York: Garland, 1985.

———. *Black Women in White: Racial Conflict and Cooperation in the Nursing Profession, 1890–1950.* Blacks in the Diaspora, edited by Darlene Clark Hine, John McCluskey Jr., and David Barry Gaspar. New York: Garland, 1989.

Hoch-Smith, Judith, and Anita Spring, eds. *Women in Ritual and Symbolic Roles.* New York: Plenum Press, 1978.

Holmes, Linda Janet. *Into the Light of Day: Reflections on the History of Midwives of Color within the American College of Nurse-Midwives.* Silver Spring, MD: Midwives of Color Committee of the American College of Nurse-Midwives, 2011.

Institute of Medicine (US). Division of Health Promotion and Disease Prevention. Committee to Study Medical Professional Liability and the Delivery of Obstetrical Care. *Medical Professional Liability and the Delivery of Obstetric Care, Volume 1.* Washington, DC: National Academy Press, 1989.

Jordan, Francis Harold. "Across the Bridge: Penn School and Penn Center." EdD diss. University of South Carolina, 1991.

Keith, Katherine L. "In Defense of Lay Midwifery: The Visual Culture of Midwife Education." *Hospital Drive.* Issue 8 (Summer 2012). http://hospitaldrive.med .virginia.edu/hospital-drive/issue-8-summer-2012/in-defense-of-lay-midwifery -the-visual-cultural-of-midwife-education/.

Ladd-Taylor, Molly. "Grannies and Spinsters: Midwife Education under the Sheppard-Towner Act." *Journal of Social History* 22, no. 2 (Winter 1988): 255–75. www.jstor.org.

Leavitt, Judith Walzer. "Joseph B. De Lee and the Practice of Preventive Obstetrics." *American Journal of Public Health* 78, no. 10 (1988): 1353–61.

——. *Brought to Bed: Childbearing in America, 1750 to 1950.* New York: Oxford University Press, 1986.

Lemann, Nicholas. *The Promised Land: The Great Black Migration and How It Changed America.* New York: Vintage Books, 1992.

Litoff, Judy Barrett. *American Midwives: 1860 to the Present.* New York: Greenwood Press, 1978.

Ludden, Forest E. *The History of Public Health in Alabama (1941–1968).* Montgomery: Alabama Department of Public Health, 1970.

McArthur, Judith N. "Maternity Wars: Gender, Race, and the Sheppard-Towner Act in Texas." University of Texas at Arlington.

Michaelson, Karen L., and contributors. *Childbirth in America: Anthropological Perspectives.* South Hadley, MA: Bergin and Garvey Publishers, 1988.

Mongeau, Beatrice, Harvey L. Smith, and Ann C. Maney. "The Granny Midwife: Changing Roles and Functions of a Folk Practitioner." *American Journal of Sociology* 66, no. 5 (1961): 497–505.

Montgomery, Warner M. "Pineville, A Historic Refuge, Part 57: Nurse Maude Is Honored." *Columbia Star,* May 2, 2008, sec. Travel.

Morgan, Marjorie. "Prenatal Care of African American Women in Selected USA Urban and Rural Cultural Contexts." *Journal of Transcultural Nursing* 7, no. 2 (January–June 1996): 3–9.

Morris, Christopher. *Becoming Southern: The Evolution of a Way of Life, Warren County and Vicksburg, Mississippi, 1770–1860.* New York: Oxford University Press, 1995.

Morton, Margaret, and Edna R. Roberts. "Celebrating Public Health Nursing: Caring for Mississippi's Communities with Courage and Compassion, 1920–1993." *Mississippi Department of Health.* http://msdh.ms.gov/msdhsite/_static/19,10778,378.html#.

Mountin, Joseph W., and Evelyn Flook. "Distribution of Health Services in the Structure of State Government: Chapter VII: Maternity-Child Health Activities by State Agencies." *Public Health Reports (1896–1970)* 57, no. 48 (1942): 1791–1821.

Murphree, A. "A Functional Analysis of Southern Folk Beliefs concerning Birth." *American Journal of Obstetrics and Gynecology* 102, no. 1 (September 1968): 125–34.

Nelson, Jennifer. "Healthcare Reconsidered: Forging Community Wellness among African Americans in the South." *Bulletin of the History of Medicine* 81, no. 3 (2007): 594–624.

Reeb, Rene M. "Granny Midwives in Mississippi: Career and Birth Practices." *Journal of Transcultural Nursing* 3, no. 2 (Winter 1992): 18–27.

Rice, Mitchell F., and Woodrow Jones Jr., eds. *Health of Black Americans from Post Reconstruction to Integration, 1871–1960.* Bibliographies and Indexes in Afro-American Studies. Vol. 26. New York: Greenwood Press, 1990.

Robinson, Sharon A. "A Historical Development of Midwifery in the Black Community: 1600–1940." *Journal of Nurse-Midwifery* 29, no. 4 (July/August 1984): 247–50.

Sandelowski, Margarete. *Pain, Pleasure, and American Childbirth: From the Twilight Sleep to the Read Method, 1914–1960*. Contributions in Medical History. Westport, CT: Greenwood Press, 1984.

Savitt, Todd L. *Race and Medicine in Nineteenth- and Early Twentieth-Century America*. Kent, OH: Kent State University Press, 2007.

Schwartz, Marie Jenkins. *Birthing a Slave: Motherhood and Medicine in the Antebellum South*. Cambridge, MA: Harvard University Press, 2009.

Shah, Mary Ann. "The Unification of Midwives: A Time for Dialogue." Journal of Nurse-Midwifery 27, no. 5 (September/October 1982): 1–2.

Shaw, Nancy Stoller. *Forced Labor: Maternity Care in the United States*. New York: Pergamon Press, 1974.

Smith, David Barton. "The Politics of Racial Disparities: Desegregating the Hospitals in Jackson, Mississippi." *Milbank Quarterly* 83, no. 2 (2005): 247–69. www.jstor.org.

Smith, Susan L. *Sick and Tired of Being Sick and Tired: Black Women's Health Activism in America, 1890–1950*. Studies in Health, Illness, and Caregiving. Edited by Joan E. Lynaugh. Philadelphia: University of Pennsylvania Press, 1995.

Stowe, Steven M. *Doctoring the South: Southern Physicians and Everyday Medicine in the Mid-Nineteenth Century*. Chapel Hill: University of North Carolina Press, 2004.

Susie, Debra Anne. *In the Way of Our Grandmothers: A Cultural View of Twentieth-Century Midwifery in Florida*. Athens: University of Georgia Press, 1988.

Thomas, Karen Kruse. *Deluxe Jim Crow: Civil Rights and American Health Policy, 1935–1954*. Athens: University of Georgia Press, 2011.

———. "The Hill-Burton Act and Civil Rights: Expanding Hospital Care for Black Southerners, 1939–1960." *Journal of Southern History* 72, no. 4 (2006): 823–70.

Townes, Emilie M. *Breaking the Fine Rain of Death: African American Health Issues and a Womanist Ethic of Care*. New York: Continuum Publishing Company, 1988.

University of Alabama Board of Trustees. "A Chronological History of the University of Alabama at Birmingham and its Predecessor Institutions and Organizations, 1831–." https://www.uab.edu/archives/chron.

Varney Burst, Helen. "History of Nurse-Midwifery in Reproductive Health Care." *Journal of Nurse Midwifery* 43, no. 6 (November–December 1998): 526–29.

Varney Burst, Helen, and Joyce Beebe Thompson. *A History of Midwifery in the United States: The Midwife Said Fear Not*. New York: Springer Publishing Company, 2015.

Ward, Thomas J., Jr. *Black Physicians in the Jim Crow South*. Fayetteville: University of Arkansas Press, 2003.

Ward, Tom. "Medical Missionaries of the Delta: Dr. Dorothy Ferebee and the Mississippi Health Project, 1935–1941." *Journal of Mississippi History* 62, no. 3 (2001): 189–203.

Warner, Geoffrey. "Racial Differences in the Hurdling of Prenatal Care Barriers." *Review of Black Political Economy* 25, no. 3 (Winter 1997): 95–114.

Washington, Harriet A. *Medical Apartheid: The Dark History of Medical Experimentation on Black Americans from Colonial Times to the Present.* New York: Anchor Books, 2006.

Wilkie, Laurie A. *The Archaeology of Mothering: An African American Midwife's Tale.* New York: Routledge, 2003.

Yang, Y. Tony, Laura B. Attanasio, and Katy B. Kozhimannil. "State Scope of Practice Laws, Nurse-Midwifery Workforce, and Childbirth Procedures and Outcome." *Women's Health Issues,* 26, no.3 (2016): 262–67. https://doi.org/10.1016/jwhi2016.02.003.

INDEX

Page numbers in **bold** refer to illustrations.

African American doctors, 96; discrimination and, 97, 99–101, 105; education, 98–100, 103, 105, 106; hospital privileges, 100–101, 103, 105; job opportunities, 99, 100
Afro-American Hospital, 102
Airhihienbuwa, Collins, 6–7
airplane midwives, 87–88
Alabama, 3, 30, 47, 72, 109–11, 121, 131, 133, 136
Amani, Jamarah, 143
Ambrose, Carol, 140
American Association of Nurse-Midwives (AANM), 91, 134
American College of Nurse-Midwives (ACNM), 123, 134, 136–37, 138–39, 140–42, 147
American Congress of Obstetrics and Gynecology, 146–47
American Medical Association, 100
Andrew Memorial Hospital, 35, 93
antibiotics, 26
Appalachia, 7–8
Arkansas, 83
asepsis, 25, 32, 34, 46, 81, 113, 114, 154n3

Bacon, Joselyn, 135, 136
Baker, J. N., 71
Barnes, Helen, 101
Baylor, Edith, 85
Beardsley, Edward, 98, 102, 115–16

Benjamin, Louvenia Taylor, 28, 29, 51, 59, 61, 129–30
Berkeley County Midwives, **85**
Best, Andrew, 113
"Birth Certificate Song," 57–58, 88
birth certificates, 33, 37, 51, 57–58, 88, 130
black hospitals, 101–2, 103, 105, 113
Blackburn, Laura, 83, 90
Bolivar County Midwives Meeting, **34**
Bolton Act, 74
Boulware, Thomas, 72, **106**, 107, 110–11, 113, 116, 148
Bousfield, M. O., 79, 103
Breckinridge, Mary, 7–8, 133–34
Broughton, Eugenia, 58–59, 74, **80**, 83, **85**, 86, 88, 89
Brown, George, 97
Bryant, Maude, 60
Bureau of Child Welfare, 33
Bureau of Vital Statistics, 57
Burst, Helen Varney, 136–37, 146

Callen, Maude, 63–64, 77, 80–81, **81**, 83, 86–87, 89, 90, **90**, 134
Charleston Birth Place, 122–23
Chicago Defender, 114
Chicago Maternity Center, 67
childbirth, 11–12, 22, 24, 41–43, 48, 60, 67, 93, 95
Children's Bureau, 24, 25, 82
Christian, Estelle W., 52
Christianity, 17
Citizens' Council, 101

Clarke, Heather, 140, 143, 144
Cody, Beatrice, 51
Coley, Mary, 46
communal vision of sickness, 17–18
Conner, Douglas, 98, 100, 101, 113
Cornley, Paul, 93, 111
cotton root, 20–21
Creanga, Andreea, 4–5
cultural empowerment model, 6–7

Davis, Michael, 116
De Lee, Joseph B., 67
Declerq, Eugene, 148
Derrell, Constance Manning, 77, 92
direct entry midwives, 11
Dorsey, Bettie, 141
doulas, 142–43, 146
Downs, Jim, 23–24
Durrell, Connie Manning, 80–81

eclampsia. See toxemia
Emergency Maternal and Infant Care pro-
    gram (EMIC), 93, 107, 108, 111, 116
eugenics, 13

Ferguson, James, 109
Fett, Sharla, 17
Fishbourne, William K., 89–90
Flint-Goodridge School, 73
Florida, 127, 129, 130–31, 133
Forte, Etta Mae, 73
Fraser, Gertrude Jacinta, 57, 93–94, 112, 118
Frontier Nursing Service, 7–8

Georgia, 21, 30, 46, 111, 127
Gewin, W. C., 25
Gibson, Faith, 115
Goan, Melanie, 134
granny midwives, 11, 27, 64, 82. See also lay
    midwives

Hagquist, Katherine, 35
Hale, Mamie O., 77, 83–84, 87–88, 90
Hamer, Fannie Lou, 48
healthcare. See maternity care

Hemschemeyer, Hattie, 134
Hicks, H. C., 53–54
Hill, J. Edward, 5–6, 135–36, 148, 149
Hill, Lillie Bell, 39, 53
Hill-Burton Act, 103, 115
Hilliard, Mary B., 30
Hines, Darlene Clark, 78
Hyder, Kate, 73

Improving Access to Maternity Care Act of
    2015, 5, 146
infant mortality rate, 4, 45, 56–57, 69, 83,
    106, 116–17, 123, 135, 137, 139, 146
integration, 9, 96, 102, 103, 104–5, 113; of
    hospitals, 4, 83
International Center for Traditional
    Childbirth (ICTC), 142, 144, 145, 147, 148
International Confederation of Midwives,
    147

Jacobi, Abraham, 69
Jarrett, Armentia, 140–41
Jefferson, Thomas, 20
John Gaston Hospital, 114
Jones, Anita M., 82
Jones, Nettie B., 92
Jones, Viola M., 53
Julius Rosenwald Fund, 73, 98, 102–3, 107

Kenney, John A., 78, 80
Kosmak, George, 68

lay midwives: advocacy for, 60–62, 121; bag,
    48, 49–50, 126; birth certificates, 33, 37,
    51, 57–58, 88, 130; changes in perception
    of, 38, 44–45, 53, 60–61; clubs, **34**, 36–38,
    39, 50, 53, 54, 84, 127–28; data collection,
    55–56; delivering for white women,
    128–29; economic status, 29–30; gift
    child, 51; government regulation of,
    9, 32–34, 36–37, 40–41, 50, 121, 125–32;
    as healers, 17–18; holistic care and, 12,
    46–47, 50–51; home demonstration pro-
    grams, 43–44, **44**, 45, 54; homes as clin-
    ics, 46–47; hygiene, 25, 30, 32, 34, 40–46,

52, 61, 81, 87, 88–89, 113, 114, 154n3; labor complications, 60; licensure, 33, 46, 49, 60, 109; macro-level care, 9, 15, 40, 46, 62, 112, 122; manual, **40, 41, 42**, 43–45, **48**, 50, 57, 60, 82, 121, 126–27; matrilineal obligation, 27–28; micro-level care, 9, 14–15, 40, 45, 46, 53, 75, 112, 115, 118–20, 121, 122; as Mother of the Church, 28–29; payment for services, 30–31; preparation for birth, 41–43; public health outreach, 36, 39, 45, 46, 47, 52–54, 75, 112; reporting families at risk, 54–55; retirement and, 127–28; spirituality of, 23, 24, 28–29, 31, 37, 39, 48, 50, 127, 132, 153n20; supervision of, 33–34, 46, 64, 70, 79, 82, 83, 85, 87, 93; termination of, 10, 14, 119, 121–22, 125–32; training of, 33–35, **36**, 39, 40, 64, 83, 84–85, 87, **87**, 88, **90**; vaccinations, 53–54, 56; white outfits, 41; working with physicians, 35, 38, 59–61, 71, 113, 130

Lee County Midwife Club, 39
licensed midwives, 11
Life magazine, 63
literacy, 86–87
Logan, Onnie Lee, 3, 10, 13, 27–28, 29–30, 40–41, 43, 45, 46, 47, 48, 49, 51, 54–55, 59, 60, 129, 130, 131–32, 145
Long, L. W., 93

Maddux, Walter H., 95
Maternal and Child Health Bureau, 135–36
maternal mortality rate, 4, 25, 26, 32, 45, 46, 47, 56–57, 71–72, 75, 83, 106, 110, 111, 112–13, 114, 116–17, 123, 139, 146, 151n5, 153n1
maternity care: access to, 3, 4–6, 9, 13, 23–24, 26–27, 47, 59–60, 67–68, 70, 72, 97, 98–99, 109–10, 120, 123, 148–49; birthing centers, 122–23, 130–31, 145; Cesarean sections, 106, 113, 137; cost of care, 30–31, 32, 97, 100, 115–16, 123, 128; cultural empowerment model, 6–7; culturally centered, 14, 71, 79, 82, 142–44, 148–49; doctor shortage,

5, 59, 62, 98–99, 109–10; economic marketplace, 128–29, 136; fear of white doctors, 13–14, 46, 48, 80; folk medicine/remedies, 20–21, 23, 24, 29, 49, 64, 97, 139; government intervention, 24, 25; home births, 115, 123, 136–37; hospital births, 25–26, 93–94, 95, 108, 109–17, 118, 121, 133, 136–37; local, 5–6; macro-level, 6–7, 8, 9, 10, 15, 40, 46, 48, 62, 64, 76, 78, 91, 94, 95, 105, 107, 108, 111, 112, 114, 115, 116, 120, 122, 133, 138–39, 143–44, 145, 147–48; micro-level, 6–7, 8, 9, 10, 14–15, 40, 45, 46, 53, 64, 68, 71, 75, 94, 107, 108, 112, 115, 116, 118–20, 121, 122, 144, 147–48; physician-managed births, 26, 93, 117; prenatal care, 5, 10, 40, 46, 47, 48, 49, 67, 69, 70, 71–72, 75, 95, 106, 109, 111, 112, 119–20, 122, 123, 128, 136, 137, 139, 146, 148–49; quality of, 25, 102–3, 111–13, 115, 120; racial disparity in, 9, 14, 25, 83, 102–3, 123, 139, 141, 145, 147; racism and, 7, 8, 26, 47, 59–60, 103–4, 111, 112, 113–14, 115, 116, 123; scientific childbirth, 26, 67, 95, 114–15, 118; in segregated hospitals, 102–3, 113–14; spirituality, 8, 139
Maternity Center Association (MCA), 67, 68, 69, 70, 71, 73, 76, 92–93, 134
Matthew, Josephine, 86
Medicaid, 4, 116, 119, 128, 129, 134, 142
midwifery: American, 10–11; changes in perception of, 38, 44–45, 53, 60–61, 69, 89–90; collaboration with physicians, 21–23, 35, 38, 59–61, 71, 88–90, 113, 130, 133, 136, 144, 146–47; diversity and, 140–44; European, 7–8, 25, 33, 68–69; government regulation, 3, 4, 9, 32–34, 36–37, 40–41, 43, 50, 67–70, 83–84, 121–23, 125–32, 134–36, 137, 143; internal issues within profession, 82, 123–24, 136–37, 144, 146, 147; legacy of, 9, 143; matrilineal obligation, 27–28; racial stereotyping and, 93–94; racism and, 9, 13, 33–34, 64, 75, 76, 91–94, 134; spirituality, 17–19, 23, 24, 28–29, 31, 37, 39, 48, 50; training for, 33–35, **36**, 39, 40, 63, 64,

65–70, 73–74, 76–81, 82–83, 84–85, 87, **87**, 88, **90**, 91–93, 106–7, 141–42, 147

Midwifery Institute, 84–85, **84**

"Midwives Song, The," 37, 85, 88–89

Midwives of Color Committee, 140–41, 143

Miller, Helen Sullivan, 76–77

Milton, Gladys, 10, 30, 59–60, 125, 129, 130–31, 132, 144

Milton, Maria, 12, 143, 145

Milton Memorial Birthing Center, 130–31, 145

Mississippi, 30, 32–33, 36, 43, 45, 52–53, 84, 101, 116, 128, 135–36

"Mississippi Appendectomy," 48

Mitchell, Matilda Holt, 44–45

Mongeau, Beatrice, 86–97

Montgomery, Jim, 98

Moore, Jennifer Crook, 3–4

Morris, Christopher, 21

motherwit, 24, 28, 118

Muhammad, JayVon, 144

Murphy, Margaret, 73, 82

National Hospital Association, 101–2

National League of Nursing, 76

National Medical Association, 101

National Organization of Public Health Nursing, 78, 79

1984 Midwifery Practice Act, 131

North Carolina, 33–35, 111

nurse-midwives: certified, 11; changes in perception of, 89–90; clinic operation, 70, 71–72, **74**, **75**, **80**; gender discrimination and, 64, 76; government regulation, 67–70, 83–84, 122–23, 134–36; macro-level care, 64, 76, 78, 91, 133, 138–39; micro-level care, 64, 71; patient relationships with, 70–71, 79, 82; professional discrimination, 64, 136; public health and, 77–78, 79, 83, 133, 138–40; racism and, 64, 76, 91–94, 134; training of, 63, 69–70, 73–74, 76–81, 82–90, 91–93, 106–7, 141–42; training/supervising lay midwives and, 64, 70, 72, 73, 79, 82, 83, 85, 87–89, **90**, 93, 133–36; unequal

pay, 92; working in places of need, 70, 74, 80–81; working with physicians, 88, 89, 133, 136

Osborne, Mary D., 32–33, 43, 83, 128

Owens, F. Carrington, 92

Peckham, Charles H., 71

Penn Center, 84–85, **85**

Phillips, Homer G., 113

plantation health care, 21–22

poverty, 3, 9, 14, 30, 40, 45–46, 49, 54, 72, 73, 81, 93, 95, 107, 111, 114, 116, 119, 128

prenatal care, 5, 10, 40, 46, 47, 48, 49, 67, 69, 70, 71–72, 75, 95, 106, 109, 111, 112, 119–20, 122, 123, 128, 136, 137, 139, 146, 148–49

prenatal clinics, 40, 47, 70, 71–72, **74**, **75**, 80, 106, 109, 111, 139, 149

Puckett, Newbell Niles, 29

racism, 8, 9, 13, 17–19, 33–34, 57, 64, 75, 76, 91–95, 97–101, 105, 107, 115, 134, 141

Rathbun, Leslie, 122–23

Reed, Mamie, 30

Reformed Episcopal Church clinic, **74**, **75**

registered midwives, 11

Reid, Jean, 32

reproduction control, 20–21

Rothert, Frances Catherine, 71–72

Savitt, Todd, 20

Schwartz, Marie Jenkins, 21

Sheppard-Towner Maternity and Infancy Act, 4, 32, 34, 43, 123

Sheriff, Hilla, 71, 83, 89

Singleton, Elizabeth, 28

slaves, 13, 17–24; forced sexual relationships, 21; gender bias, 18–19; healers and, 17–19, 23; menstruation, 20–21; midwives, 21–23; racism and, 17–18; reproduction/fertility of, 19–21; selective breeding of, 21; soundness of, 19; spirituality, 17–19, 23

Slossfield Community Center, 105–6

Slossfield Medical Center, 95, 106–7, **108**, 110, 113
Smith, Claudine Curry, 10, 27, 30, 31, 45–46, 51, 59, 60, 61, 115, 119, 130
Smith, Margaret Charles, 3, 10, 21, 27, 28, 30, **31**, 45, 46, 47, 59, 61, 115, 118, 120, 126, 130, 131, 145
Smith, Rosie, 50
Smith, W. Eugene, 63, 80–81
socialized medicine, 110, 116
"Song of the Midwives," 54
South Carolina, 57, 63, **81**, 82–87, **84**, **85**, 107, 109, 111, 116–17, 119, 122–23, 128, 136
South Carolina Medical Association, 123
Southern Rural Black Women's Initiative (SRBWI), 3–4, 5
St. Martin de Porres Hospital, 114
Staggers, Ruker, 61, 130, 131
Stokes, Mamie, 85

Thomas, Margaret, 73–74, 92
toxemia (eclampsia), 46, 114
Trabert, Lois, 35

Trammel, Beatrice, 74
Travis, John, 21
Tuskegee, Alabama, 35
Tuskegee School of Nurse-Midwifery, 63, 73–74, 76–77, 78–79, 83–84, 91–93

Underwood, Felix, 35, 36, 38, 45, 54, 60–61, 78, 83
United States Midwifery Education, Regulation and Association (US MERA), 144, 147

vaccinations, 53–54, 56
Van Blarcom, Carolyn Conant, 68–69

Walker, Clara, 23
Ward, Thomas J., 100
Washington, Harriet, 48
Watson, Benjamin P., 68
Watson, Edwin R., 71
Weston, Randy, 101
White-Walker, Shirley, 140

Printed in the United States
By Bookmasters